ADDRESSING PATIENTS' HEALTH LITERACY NEEDS

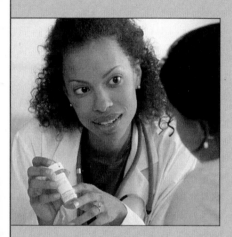

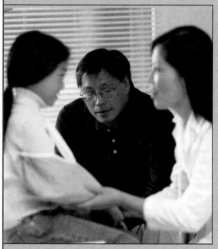

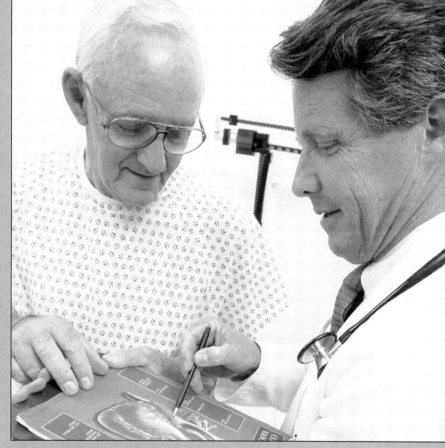

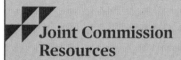
Joint Commission Resources

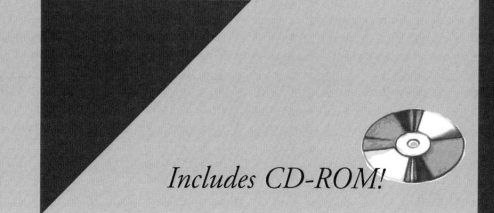
Includes CD-ROM!

Senior Editor: Robert A. Porché, Jr.
Senior Project Manager: Cheryl Firestone
Associate Director, Production: Johanna Harris
Associate Director, Editorial Development: Diane Bell
Executive Director: Catherine Chopp Hinckley, Ph.D.
Vice President, Learning: Charles J. Macfarlane, F.A.C.H.E.
Joint Commission/JCR Reviewers: Diane Bell, Erica Galvez, Michael Kulczycki, Carol Mooney, Amy Wilson-Stronks, Debra Zak, Gina Zimmerman

Joint Commission Resources Mission
The mission of Joint Commission Resources (JCR) is to continuously improve the safety and quality of health care in the United States and in the international community through the provision of education, publications, consultation, and evaluation services.

Joint Commission Resources educational programs and publications support, but are separate from, the accreditation activities of The Joint Commission. Attendees at Joint Commission Resources educational programs and purchasers of Joint Commission Resources publications receive no special consideration or treatment in, or confidential information about, the accreditation process.

The inclusion of an organization name, product, or service in a Joint Commission Resources publication should not be construed as an endorsement of such organization, product, or service, nor is failure to include an organization name, product, or service to be construed as disapproval.

Requests for permission to make copies of any part of this work should be mailed to
Permissions Editor
Department of Publications
Joint Commission Resources
One Renaissance Boulevard
Oakbrook Terrace, Illinois 60181
permissions@jcrinc.com

ISBN: 978-1-59940-280-2
Library of Congress Control Number: 2009922544

For more information about Joint Commission Resources, please visit http://www.jcrinc.com.

CONTENTS

INTRODUCTION

Far too often, patients experience confusion, frustration, miscommunication, or a preventable adverse event in their interactions with health care providers. Could these barriers to quality health care have been avoided if the communication gap between patients and caregivers was tightened? Certainly, statistics show that a significant number of adverse events can be attributed to low health literacy levels in patients. When patients do not understand medical jargon and procedures, or cannot read health care documentation, they are less likely to understand when a process might be wrong, or they may be afraid to speak up when they suspect something is not right. The consequences of limited health literacy go beyond preventable adverse health care events. They can include financial repercussions, increased ER/physician visits, insurance issues, care accessibility issues, and poor health behavior choices.

What can the health care community do to bridge this gap? Perhaps the first step in fixing the problem lies with health care providers first understanding what is included under the umbrella of inadequate health literacy, what the origins of illiteracy may be, and what strategies to overcome health literacy issues may be most effective.

Addressing Patients' Health Literacy Needs focuses on health literacy as it affects patient safety and health care outcomes. This book thoroughly examines the health literacy crisis in the United States and provides effective techniques for improving the health literacy of patients and bridging the communication gap between caregivers and patients.

Chapter 1 details the many elements that contribute to health literacy and how the health care system is currently unable to meet most of the needs of a population in which low literacy, poor English skills, and other constraints are becoming the norm rather than the exception. There is also an explanation of how poor health literacy leads to poor health outcomes, patient safety issues, an inefficient use of health care resources,

limited access to care, and serious economic consequences for the nation as a whole. Finally, the chapter summarizes some of the actions both public and private organizations are taking to try to address the many problems related to low health literacy.

In Chapter 2, you will find descriptions of populations who are at high risk for poor health literacy, as well as ways to recognize those who may be having trouble understanding instructions and explanations of care— even if they do not belong to a high-risk group. These methods include verbal and nonverbal clues from the patient and, if you are trying to identify the needs of a specific group, standardized tests that can help you tailor your activities. There is also a section on the importance of collecting data both before and after you attempt to make improvements to processes and materials so you can judge the effectiveness of interventions.

Chapter 3 contains suggestions of ways to address poor health literacy and the need to make these activities an organizationwide priority that involves all employees and staff. The techniques included here cover effective ways to improve everything from patient education materials to the signage in your organization to verbal communication with patients and family members.

The suggestions from the previous chapter come to life in Chapter 4, which contains seven case studies from real organizations. You will see how individual facilities, large systems, and statewide entities have found ways to incorporate methods such as teach-back, "Ask Me 3™," and simplified informed consent to help their populations better understand and participate in their own care. You will also find examples of how staff of all levels and disciplines can be educated about health literacy and how patients' contributions to developing processes and materials increases success.

Finally, the appendix gives you a modest compendium of resources to help you further investigate the problems and possible solutions for low health literacy.

The brief glossary that ends this book provides definitions for many terms related to health literacy.

Addressing Patients' Health Literacy Needs also features an accompanying CD-ROM. This component offers a collection of informational resources designed to enhance and expand upon the book's content. Among other features, the disk includes all seven case studies presented in Chapter 4 of this publication.

A Note on Terminology
This book is intended to help a variety of health care organizations—including hospital, ambulatory care, behavioral health care, long term care, and home care organizations—address health literacy issues. Because each setting has its own terminology, the text uses the following terms generically throughout:

➤ *Patient*—Anyone receiving care, treatment, or services from an organization, including residents (long term care), individuals being served (behavioral health care), members (networks and preferred provider organizations,) and clients (home care)

➤ *Staff members*—Individuals who work within a health care organization, including administrative, clinical and nonclinical care, and support staff members

➤ *Family*—Those who play a significant role in a patient's life and who form a social support system for that patient. This can include people who are not legally related to the patient as well.

➤ *Care*—Clinical and nonclinical interventions (care, treatment, or services)

➤ *Health care organization*—Any facility that delivers care, treatment, or services, including ambulatory care centers, assisted living facilities, behavioral health organizations (residential and nonresidential), home care agencies, hospitals, and long term care institutions

ACKNOWLEDGMENTS
Joint Commission Resources wishes to acknowledge the contributions of the various individuals, health care organizations, and health systems that shared their outstanding case studies, examples, and program materials for this book. These individuals and organizations include the following:
➤ Marge Kars, M.L.S., A.H.I.P., Manager, Bronson Health Sciences Library and Bronson HealthAnswers, Bronson Methodist Hospital, Kalamazoo, Michigan

➤ Dr. Sunil Kripalani, M.D., M.Sc., Chief, Section of Hospital Medicine, Vanderbilt Center for Health Services Research, Nashville, Tennessee

➤ Grady Health System, Department of Multicultural Affairs, Atlanta

➤ Mary Ann Abrams, M.D., M.P.H., Clinical Performance Improvement, Iowa Health System, Des Moines

➤ Robert Moravec, M.D., Medical Director, St. Joseph's Hospital, St. Paul; The Minnesota Hospital Association, St. Paul

➤ Tania Daniels and Christine Norton, The Minnesota Hospital Association, St. Paul

➤ Lane Stiles, director, Fairview Press, Minneapolis

➤ H. Shonna Yin, M.D., M.S., Department of Pediatrics, New York University School of Medicine, New York City

➤ Linda van Schaick, M.S.Ed., The HELP Project, Bellevue Hospital Center, New York City

➤ Virginia S. Tong, M.S.W., Vice President, Cultural Competence, Lutheran HealthCare, Brooklyn, New York

Thanks are also extended to Terry Davis, Department of General-Internal Medicine, Louisiana State University Health Sciences Center, School of Medicine, Shreveport; Ann Laramee, Clinical Nurse Specialist, Cardiology, and Nurse Practitioner, Heart Failure Clinic, Fletcher Allen Health Care, Burlington, Vermont; and Urmimala Sarkar, University of California, San Francisco.

Finally, we reserve our greatest debt of gratitude to Karen Steib for her excellent job of writing this publication.

CHAPTER 1
UNDERSTANDING HEALTH LITERACY

No kidney stones are identified. The right kidney is somewhat malrotated. There is a somewhat vague area of increased attenuation at the midpole medially in the right kidney that could be a high-density cyst.

—A preliminary diagnostic report from a computed tomography scan

Some people are sensitive to the following, which can lower blood sugar: tobacco, caffeine, and certain medicines such as aspirin, haloperidol, propoxyphene, chlorpromazine, (propanolol, and disopyramid). If you are taking any of these medicines, contact your physician to discuss alternative prescriptions.

—Discharge instructions for hypoglycemia after emergency department treatment

Any amounts showing in the deductible and coinsurance columns represent amounts applied to your out-of-pocket maximum. The amount in the Other Amounts Not Covered column represent your total liability for this claim.

—Explanation of benefits for a Medicare supplement

Patients constantly receive materials with this type of language from health care providers and third-party payers. Unfortunately, a large number of the people who try to read such materials will not understand them. According to the Agency for Healthcare Research and Quality (AHRQ), only 12% of 228 million adult Americans have the skills necessary to manage their own health care competently.[1] People of all ages, races, income levels, and educational backgrounds are challenged by poor health literacy. Admission and consent forms, appointment cards, explanations of diagnoses, educational materials, insurance and billing statements, and instructions for medications are just some of the hurdles that individuals with low health literacy must overcome when they enter the health care continuum. These hurdles can be so daunting that many people choose not to attempt them, opting to avoid medical advice or treatment until health problems become so severe that they demand immediate attention.

The need for adequate health literacy has grown and has been complicated by the increasing complexity of clinical interventions and of the health care system itself. Although ever-expanding technology makes new treatments possible, it is more difficult to explain these treatment options to patients who may have trouble with a basic understanding of their disease or condition, let alone the terminology inherent in descriptions of complex medical procedures. Patients, particularly those with chronic diseases, must accept more responsibility for self-care, which involves monitoring vital signs, medication regimens, and dietary restrictions—activities that require skills beyond those that many people use in their daily lives.

Defining Health Literacy

Both the Institute of Medicine (IOM) and the American Medical Association (AMA) define *health literacy* as "the ability to obtain, process, and understand basic health information and services needed to make appropriate health decisions and follow instructions for treatment." However, the IOM's 2004 report *Health Literacy: A Prescription to End Confusion* notes that "health literacy goes beyond the individual. It also depends upon the skills, preferences, and expectations of health information and care providers: our doctors, nurses, administrators, home health workers, the media, and many others."[2]

The definition developed for the National Library of Medicine and found on the Web sites of both Healthy People 2010 (http://www.healthypeople.gov) and the American College of Physicians (ACP) Foundation (http://foundation.acponline.org) is similar: "the degree to which individuals have the capacity to obtain, process, and understand basic health information and services needed to make appropriate decisions."

Sociolinguist Christina Zarcadoolas, Ph.D., and colleagues take this theme a step further, stating that a person with good health literacy can discuss topics such as health and scientific knowledge; that health literacy evolves over the course of a person's life; and that it is affected by factors such as a person's health, demographics, psychosocial status, and culture. They define health literacy as "the wide range of skills and competencies that people develop to seek out, comprehend, evaluate, and use health information and concepts to make informed choices, reduce health risks, and increase quality of life."[3] Table 1-1 (right) lists some of the myriad aspects of a person's life that can affect his or her health literacy level.

Whatever definition you use, health literacy has many levels and is influenced by the composite of a person's life. The following are some of the levels that have been recognized:

➤ **Basic/functional/fundamental health literacy:** using the basic skills of reading, writing, and numeracy to complete everyday tasks, including making and keeping appointments and following directions on medication labels[3-5]

➤ **Communicative/interactive health literacy:** having both the social skills and the more advanced cognitive and literacy skills to be able to actively participate in one's own care, find and understand information, and apply that information to one's current situation[4]

➤ **Science literacy:** Understanding scientific concepts, technology, and the rapid changes that take place in this field[3]

Table 1-1. Factors That Influence Level of Health Literacy

General		
■ Age	■ Education	■ Race/ethnicity

Physical		
■ Vision	■ Hearing	■ Verbal ability
■ Memory	■ Reasoning	

Social		
■ Occupation	■ Employment	■ Income
■ Social support	■ Culture	■ Language

➤ **Civic literacy:** being aware of public issues, including civic and governmental processes, and how individual health decisions can affect public health[3]

➤ **Cultural literacy:** interpreting and using health information based on one's beliefs, customs, and so on[3]

➤ **Critical health literacy:** using advanced social and cognitive skills to critically analyze information and to use this information to exert greater control over one's health and circumstances[4]

Levels of health literacy can also be specific to different types of conditions. For example, a person's knowledge and beliefs about mental illness indicate his or her *mental health literacy*. Those with poor mental health literacy usually cannot accurately identify common mental disorders and believe that emotional problems either will go away on their own or should be solved without help from outsiders. This can lead to delays in diagnosis and treatment, as well as attempts to use less effective treatments as self-treatment.[6] There is also *maternal health literacy*, defined as "the cognitive and social skills that determine the motivation and ability of women to gain access to, understand, and use information in ways that promote and maintain their health and that of their children."[7]

According to the Joint Committee on National Health Education Standards, a health-literate person is a critical thinker and problem solver, a responsible and productive citizen, a self-directed learner, and an effective communicator.[8] However, one's health literacy

Table 1-2. Health Literacy Levels and Abilities from National Assessment of Adult Literacy Results

Level	% of Respondents	Description	Sample Survey Tasks
1. Below basic	14%	Unable to perform basic tasks	▪ Reading a short set of instructions to identify what a patient can drink before a specific test ▪ Signing a form
2. Basic	22%	Can perform basic tasks involved with reading and understanding clearly presented health information, but has difficulty comprehending typical patient education materials or filling out insurance forms	▪ Reading a pamphlet to identify two reasons an asymptomatic person should be screened for a specific disease ▪ Reading a two-page article on a chronic medical condition and explaining why people often don't know they have this condition
3. Intermediate	53%	Can handle most prose and numerical information encountered in a health care setting, but would have trouble with complex documents	▪ Figuring out dosing times for a prescription drug based on the label's instructions to take the drug with food ▪ Consulting reference materials to determine which foods contain a certain vitamin
4. Proficient	13%	Can read and understand almost all information they may encounter in a health care setting	▪ Interpreting a table about blood pressure, age, and physical activity ▪ Determining an employee's share of annual health insurance costs from a table showing the monthly costs of different plans

Sources: Kutner M., et al.: *The Health Literacy of America's Adults: Results from the 2003 National Assessment of Adult Literacy.* (NCES 2006-483). Washington, DC: U.S. Department of Education, National Center for Education Statistics, 2006; Partnership for Clear Health Communication: *What Is Health Literacy?* 2006. http://www.npsf.org/pchc/health-literacy.php (accessed Feb. 15, 2009).

levels vary according to one's situation. Those with little education, poor English skills, or cognitive disabilities may not be able to communicate effectively or may not be motivated to educate themselves about health topics such as preventive care and diagnostics. Even individuals who hold jobs that demand excellent reading and critical thinking skills can be confused by information that contains unfamiliar medical jargon or the need to navigate a health system they have never used beyond an occasional visit to their primary care physicians.

"We need a health literate America," says Ruth Parker, M.D., Professor of Medicine at Emory University. "We need a population in this country that understands what they need to do to take care of their health. [Health] literacy really is about functioning; it's not just about reading and writing. Can you access and use information to function? The number of people who struggle with that is astounding."[9]

The Growing Problem

Although health literacy is influenced by far more than

general literacy level, reading, writing, and arithmetic are still the main building blocks for other skills, such as critical thinking. Unfortunately, the levels of adult literacy in the United States are alarmingly low.

The 2003 National Assessment of Adult Literacy (NAAL) tested a random sample of 19,000 adults from across the country to measure reading and comprehension, document interpretation, and numeracy. Some of the items in the survey were aimed at evaluating health literacy, focusing on scenarios such as preventing and treating illness and navigating the health care system. Survey results were divided into four basic categories: (1) below basic, (2) basic, (3) intermediate, and (4) proficient (*see* Table 1-2, page 3). Although 53% of the population performed at the intermediate level, meaning those individuals can read and understand most of the information they are given in a health care encounter, 22% had only basic health literacy skills, and an additional 14% had even lower results.[10] People in the two latter groups find it difficult or impossible to understand traditional explanations of diagnoses and treatment options; discharge instructions or self-care regimens; or requests for information beyond their name, address, and birth date on a medical history form.

The NAAL data also showed that 11 million adults are nonliterate in English.[10] Evidence of the problem surfaced in the 1990s, when researchers for the National Adult Literacy Survey (NALS) interviewed more than 26,000 adults age 16 and over to determine their performance levels in prose literacy (understanding running text such as brochures or news stories), document literacy (finding and using information presented in other formats such as tables and charts), and numeracy (performing calculations and understanding mathematical concepts). Results showed that approximately 20% of the population had poor skills in all three areas (Level 1), whereas 25%–28%, or 50 million people, were only slightly above that (Level 2).[11] Although many adults age 65 and over thought they had no problems with literacy, the survey found that most scored in the two lowest literacy levels in all three categories: 71% for prose literacy, 80% for document literacy, and 68% for numeracy.[12]

The International Adult Literacy Survey (IALS), which was conducted between 1994 and 1998, determined the literacy levels of people in 22 industrialized, high-income countries. The overall scores for American adults were ranked as average when compared to those for the other countries, but when the scores were broken down based on demographics, certain disparities were found. For example, there were larger differences in literacy levels between various U.S. populations than between those in other countries (nonwhite racial groups in the United States scored significantly below European Americans.) The average scores for young adults were also below those of their peers in other countries who had comparable levels of education and income.[13,14]

Looking at the tasks used in the NALS and the IALS to determine general literacy, researchers identified 191 topics that were health related—such as first aid, disease prevention and treatment, drugs and alcohol, safety and accident prevention, wellness, and emergency care—and created the Health Activities Literacy Scale to analyze the health literacy of U.S. adults. The health literacy skills of approximately 12% of Americans were at the lowest level (performing simple acts such as keeping appointments), and 7% more were even lower. Almost 50% of adults who hadn't completed high school ranked in the lowest health literacy level, as did nearly 50% of adults 65 and over.[15]

Even more disturbing than the historical data are current predictions for the future. The title of a 2007 report from the Educational Testing Service, *America's Perfect Storm,* refers to the imminent national epidemic of low health literacy. After surveying the current state of literacy skills, the report predicted that the average skills of adults age 16 to 65 years will decline significantly by 2030. More people will have trouble or be unable to handle basic health-related tasks, such as understanding medication instructions and consent forms. The average literacy skills of the elderly are expected to decline even more. The report cites several reasons for this problem, including a high school graduation rate of only 70%, with a lack of any significant improvement in high school reading and math performance, particularly among African American and Hispanic students. The major shift in U.S. demographics, with immigrants expected to make up more than half of the nation's population growth by 2015, also contributes to poor literacy because many of these individuals have less than a high school education, and the majority do not speak English. The economy is also a deciding factor; well-educated workers will retire and be replaced by those with more limited skills, making competition for well-paying jobs (with commensurate health benefits) more intense.[16]

The problems for non-English-speaking populations are not limited to the United States. The 2003 International Adult Literacy and Skills Survey—a follow-up to the 1994 IALS—tested more than 23,000 Canadians age 16 and over for proficiency in prose literacy, document literacy, numeracy, and problem solving. Even when income and education levels are the same, French-speaking Canadians (outside Quebec) tended to have lower scores than their English-speaking counterparts.[17] About 48% of adults over 16 scored at the two lowest levels for prose literacy, and 55% were at those same levels for numeracy. The survey also included questions for self-reporting physical and mental health. Respondents between 16 and 65 who reported being in poor physical health also scored lower in document literacy than did those who reported being in better health.[18]

Given the greater educational needs of people with low health literacy, the health care system as a whole seems unprepared to meet them. Outside the acute care setting, the job of educating patients often falls to physicians, nurses, and therapists because the cost of trained educators can be prohibitive. However, training in communication, health disparities, and health literacy is often inadequate in the education of health professionals. Physicians who are limited to 15 minutes with each patient are often hard-pressed to find the time to ensure they've elicited all relevant information, garnered a patient's understanding of their explanations, or provided education. Even in hospitals, staffing and budget shortfalls can mean cutbacks in patient education, leaving fewer educators and fewer resources to revise or develop materials for vulnerable and at-risk populations.

On a corporate level, health care organizations can also find themselves with competing priorities. Where there are limited resources and limited time, the necessity of health literacy is trumped by even more pressing patient needs. The organization's commitment defaults to issues like infection control or medication reconciliation. More pressing issues like these move to the top of the list, relegating things like cultural competence or health literacy toward the bottom.

The Impact of Poor Health Literacy

The limitations imposed on providers represent an important barrier to improving health literacy, but so too is a lack of awareness. Many health care professionals do not understand what a serious detriment low health literacy is to their patients, and some leaders do not understand what a serious problem it is for their organization. For example, a California study of hospital executives found that although 65% of interviewees knew of the correlation between low health literacy and medical errors, only 25% thought it was a high enough priority to be addressed.[19] Low health literacy affects not only the individual, who may not present for treatment in time or may be unable to follow self-care instructions, but also health care facilities and insurers (sicker patients require more resources) and the general population (poor lifestyle choices can affect public health, and inefficient use of medical resources drives up insurance premiums).

Poor Health Outcomes

Poor health outcomes are usually expressed in terms of mortality, morbidity, disability, dysfunction, quality of life, and functional independence.[4] For example, a 2008 study by the American Cancer Society found that death rates for Americans with high levels of education dropped significantly between 1993 and 2001, but those for people with the least amount of education went up.[20] Research conducted in U.S. hospitals by The Joint Commission found differences in the type and outcome of adverse events occurring among limited English proficient (LEP) and English-speaking patients. Some type of physical harm was involved in 49.2% of LEP individuals who reported such events, whereas the rate was 29.5% for those who spoke English. Permanent/severe harm or death occurred in 3.7% of LEP patients but in only 1.4% of English speakers. Causes for these disparities may be related to the LEP patients' inability to communicate concerns or responses, understand new information given by staff, or fully participate in their care.[21]

Since 2000 a variety of studies have been conducted to determine whether and how health literacy level affects overall health. Results showed that people with poor health literacy reported being in poorer health than those with higher levels[2] and were also more likely to be hospitalized, use emergency services, leave the hospital against medical advice, miss follow-up appointments, not have a regular physician or knowledge of their disease, and experience poor health outcomes.[22–24]

A 2007 study identified inadequate health literacy, measured by reading fluency, as a good predictor of all-cause mortality and cardiovascular death. In 1997 researchers interviewed 3,260 Medicare managed-care enrollees in four U.S. metropolitan areas about their chronic conditions, self-reported physical and mental health, and health behaviors. Demographic characteristics were noted, and the short version of the Test of Functional Health Literacy in Adults (discussed in Chapter 2) was administered to determine health literacy levels. Ten years later, the researchers studied the mortality rates of these patients: It was 18.9% for participants with "adequate" literacy, 28.7% for those with "marginal" literacy, and 39.4% for those with an "inadequate" rating.[25]

People with chronic illnesses have many opportunities to experience poor outcomes due to low health literacy. If they cannot make themselves understood when explaining symptoms or cannot get clear, reliable information about their condition, they may become frustrated and decide to forgo treatment altogether.[21] Following complex care plans correctly can be challenging even for health-literate patients. For example, people with HIV need to follow treatment regimens meticulously to slow disease progression, but those with low literacy may need special education and follow-up to understand the importance of compliance. Researchers who surveyed and interviewed 339 HIV–infected men

and women found that nearly 25% had limited health literacy, as demonstrated by the struggle to understand simple medical instructions. The patients also had lower CD4+ cell counts and higher HIV RNA levels, were less likely to take antiretroviral medications, and reported more hospitalizations and poorer general health than those with higher literacy levels.[26]

Daily activities that people with conditions such as diabetes, hypertension, or heart disease need to perform to monitor and maintain health may also be beyond the capabilities of someone with low health literacy. For example, many try to follow the written instructions that come with a glucose meter or blood pressure cuff, but they need one-on-one education from a health professional to understand how to use the instrument. Even with additional education, they may not be able to interpret the numbers on the readings correctly.

Even common diagnostic procedures can pose difficulties. Patients with limited health literacy may not understand instructions for fasting or other preparatory measures, leading to postponement of the procedures or incorrect results that can either suggest an incorrect treatment plan or necessitate repetition of the test. Individuals may also have trouble scheduling and keeping follow-up appointments, increasing the chances of a potentially serious illness being left untreated. For example, out of 538 women who were screened for health literacy while they were waiting for Pap smears, only one third who had abnormal results went through with recommended follow-up procedures. The rate of failed follow-up among patients with low health literacy was about 13 times higher than that of patients with adequate literacy.[27]

Compliance with any type of care regimen can be difficult for patients with poor health literacy, but the area of medication use carries even more risks than most. Many physicians and nurses have stories about generally literate individuals who have not administered medications properly—using pills as suppositories or taking suppositories as pills—in the latter case, even neglecting to remove the foil covering. Low-literacy patients may be unable to read or interpret the instructions on medication bottles or to comprehend verbal instructions from health professionals, meaning they do not understand dosing times, how to avoid food or drug interactions, what side effects should be reported, or how to take the drug. They also may misunderstand, distrust, or doubt the need for a physician's or health care team's plan of care and deliberately stop taking medications or take less than has been prescribed.[24,28] Medication errors are frighteningly common when parents with low health literacy try to give their children drugs. They may not be able to determine the correct dosage of cough syrup, correctly prepare an albuterol inhaler or oral rehydration solution, or administer insulin correctly.[29] Because dosing for many children's medicines is based on weight, an error can easily lead to an overdose.

Poor Behavior Choices

In addition to having trouble with tasks directly associated with health outcomes, people with limited health literacy often have less knowledge of anatomy, how disease spreads, and why early screening is important.[30] Again, anecdotes from nurses, physicians, nutritionists, and others illustrate how a lack of understanding can lead to behaviors that ultimately threaten good health. For example, there is the 25-year-old woman who thinks she is protected from sexually transmitted diseases because she takes birth control pills. Or the seriously overweight, 40-year-old man who describes himself as "husky" and eats a high-fat, high-cholesterol diet, making no connection between the chest pains he sometimes feels, his eating habits and sedentary lifestyle, and the fact that his father died of a heart attack at 49. Or the immigrant Chinese couple who do not believe their baby daughter requires the immunizations their pediatrician recommends. Individuals may engage in any number of risky behaviors—including smoking, overeating, substance abuse, and excessive alcohol consumption—simply because they do not know they can be harmed or do not believe that the risks apply to them.

Health literacy is necessary not only to avoid poor behaviors, but to engage in healthy ones. Studies have shown a statistically significant association between high health literacy levels and knowledge/use of the following preventive services[23,24,31]:

- ➤ Cervical cancer screening
- ➤ Colorectal cancer screening
- ➤ Mammography
- ➤ Prostate cancer screening

Researchers have suggested that for individuals to agree to cancer screening they must believe that it is possible for them to get the disease, that a late-stage diagnosis would have serious health consequences, and that there is something they can do to protect themselves. However, people with low health literacy may not have the information or understanding to hold these beliefs, so they avoid screening.[32]

Increased Use of Inpatient and Emergency Care

Because people with poor health literacy usually do not make use of preventive care and screening options such as flu shots and HIV testing, they usually do not seek help until their conditions are serious and they have to rely on emergency care.[22,33] The inability to interpret directions for over-the-counter and prescription drugs can lead to medication errors that require immediate intervention, as can a lack of self-care for chronic diseases such as asthma, diabetes, and heart disease. Others use the emergency department in lieu of a primary care physician.

People with poor health literacy also have a 29% to 69% higher rate of hospitalization[34] and tend to stay in the hospital about two days longer than those with better health literacy skills.[35]

Difficulties in Accessing Care

Finding a physician, navigating a clinic or hospital, providing a medical history, figuring out insurance coverage—all of these can be challenging enough for the health literate. They are particularly intimidating for someone with limited health literacy. Access to care and health information is a serious problem, particularly for LEP patients. People who are uncomfortable speaking English are less likely to have regular sources of medical care (such as a family physician or a community clinic), seek emergency care, fill prescriptions, or visit a dentist.[36]

One study found that insured Latinos with limited English skills experienced longer wait times and had more difficulty obtaining information or advice by phone than insured Latinos who were English proficient. The same held true for Latino patients on Medicare or Medicaid.[37]

Many individuals may not know how to apply for Medicaid or state health plans, and people without reliable health insurance are far less likely to use health care services and are thus less experienced at navigating the system. Of the respondents in the 2003 NAAL, 28% of those at the lowest health literacy level and 25% of those at the basic level had no insurance.[38] Researchers have shown that 18% of English-speaking and 49% of Spanish-speaking patients at two public hospitals could not understand the rights and responsibilities section of the Medicaid application form. This section contains the informed consent that patients must give to obtain financial assistance, and those with low literacy may have less access to Medicaid because they do not understand what is required.[39] Most insurance application forms are written at the 10th-grade level or higher, with dense copy, long pages, and complicated questions.[21]

Low-income and LEP families are not the only ones who contend with the financial challenges of accessing necessary health care. With the ever-rising cost of premiums, more and more people in middle income brackets are being forced to forgo insurance so they can pay mortgages, auto and school loans, and everyday expenses. As major corporations and small businesses decrease the amount of their contributions to employee health plans and cut out all health benefits to retirees and spouses, many people find they can no longer afford the wellness screenings, regular physician visits, and medications they previously took for granted. Older adults who once had employer-paid Medicare supplements and prescription coverage have trouble paying for those supplements and purchasing medications on fixed incomes. Although the phenomenon of dwindling coverage is widespread, many patients are reluctant to admit to their clinicians that cost has become a determining factor in how they manage their health care—or in many cases, whether they seek care at all. As a result, they attempt to self-diag-nose and self-treat based on information they find on the Internet or on advice from family and friends, but many do not have sufficient health literacy to determine what sources are reliable, what the risks involved in self-medicating with various over-the-counter supplements and drugs are, or when professional medical care is crucial.

Economic Issues

Costs incurred by patients with low health literacy are estimated to be much higher than those associated with health-literate individuals. Results from a small study of Medicaid managed-care enrollees showed that those at higher literacy levels generated an average $2,891 in annual health care costs, whereas those with a reading level at or below third grade generated an average of $10,688.[40]

Individuals are not the only ones to pay the price for poor health literacy. The higher number of hospitalizations, excessive use of emergency care, medication errors, and higher acuity of illness due to poor self-care costs the U.S. health care system billions of dollars each year. Although the numbers vary among studies, they are uniformly staggering. Some reports put the annual cost of low health literacy at $58 billion.[41] According to the National Academy on an Aging Society, low health literacy levels increase health care expenditures by more than $73 billion a year. Patients' out-of-pocket expenditures total more than $11 billion of literacy-related costs. Medicare pays 39% of these costs, Medicaid pays 14%, and employers as much as 17%, but most of the burden is passed on to taxpayers.[42]

Cultural Issues

Patient-provider communication is influenced by a wide variety of factors. At a time when health care facilities and private practices are serving increasingly diverse patient populations, cultural competence is still a problem in many areas. Health literacy is influenced by a person's entire belief system, based on family background, religion, ethnicity, social standing, values, and so on. When providers fail to take these factors into account or when they see patients of different nationalities and incomes as stereotypes, trust is eroded. Patients who feel they have been snubbed or treated in a condescending manner by health professionals may be less likely to follow medical advice or seek it in the future.

Failure to identify the language needs of patients is also problematic. With more than 300 languages being spoken across the country, interpreter services are in high demand, but many practitioners still do not see the need for them. They do not question a patient who says he or she can understand English; if that patient's skills are only rudimentary, the odds of him or her understanding a diagnosis or an informed consent discussion are minimal.

Many health professionals also suffer from the misconception that the only people at risk for limited health literacy are those who are poor, have a low level of education, do not speak English, or have some mental or physical liabilities. This makes it more difficult for people who do not fit into one or more of these categories to admit that they need help finding, understanding, and/or using health information. Skilled workers and highly educated professionals feel that they should be able to understand medical jargon simply because they can understand the language of their own jobs. People in middle or upper income brackets do not want to risk the stigma attached to not being able to read or calculate well. Older people worry about being viewed as incapable of handling their own affairs and living independently.

No matter what the reason, the reluctance or inability of patients and health professionals to recognize poor health literacy makes it even more difficult for organizations to address the problem.

What Is Being Done to Solve the Problem

With the dilemma of poor health literacy continuing to grow and affect every part of the health care system, stakeholders throughout this system have begun to recognize that they must participate in finding solutions. All types of health care organizations, health plans and insurers, pharmacies and pharmaceutical companies, public health agencies, patient advocacy groups, community health centers, literacy groups, professional associations—in short, anyone who provides health information and/or care—are responsible for ensuring that their information is clear and understandable.[43] This section discusses only some of the activities that have taken place to date; many more exist or are in the planning stage.

The Joint Commission's Position

Communication problems are the most frequent root cause of serious adverse events reported to The Joint Commission's Sentinel Event Database. The Joint Commission first developed standards requiring health care organizations to address a patient's language needs based on the patient's right to be fully informed about his or her care. However, the issue of effective communication has since expanded with the knowledge that it is necessary to provide the best possible care. The following principles guide The Joint Commission's approach to removing communication barriers related to language; cultural differences; low health literacy; and physical conditions such as hearing, vision, and speech impairment[44]:

➤ Providing safe, high-quality patient care depends on effective communication between health care professionals, patients, and families.

➤ To establish this type of communication, organizations and staff must recognize and work to eliminate language barriers, misunderstanding caused by cultural differences, and low health literacy.

➤ A growing body of evidence-based practices addresses these problems, and there is evidence that certain practices are ineffective or unsafe.

➤ For practices to be implemented effectively and reliably and sustained over time, they should be incorporated into an organization's work processes.

➤ Because process changes can lead to unintended consequences, organizations should proactively assess revised processes for possible problems and monitor performance after they are implemented.

Current Joint Commission accreditation standards for all programs require that a patient's language and communication be included in the medical record; that organizations provide effective communication, which includes taking health literacy issues into account; and that patient education be carried out in a way that meets the patient's communication and learning needs, whether this necessitates the use of an interpreter or sign language, appropriate visual aids, or some other method. The Joint Commission, with funding from The Commonwealth Fund, is currently developing hospital accreditation standards to promote, facilitate, and advance the delivery of culturally competent, patient-centered care, which should also help issues of health literacy related to cultural and language differences.

Although the National Patient Safety Goals—program-specific accreditation requirements established by a panel of patient safety experts—do not specifically address health literacy, several are related to communication issues that can be exacerbated when patients have limited health literacy. For example, it can be difficult to encourage patients to participate in their own care when they cannot understand the medical jargon used in explanations of diagnoses and treatment options. Even accurate identification of a patient can be problematic if he or she does not speak English or has cognitive impairments.[45]

Along with the Centers for Medicare & Medicaid Services, The Joint Commission launched a national campaign in 2002 to encourage patients to become active and informed participants in their own care and help prevent possible health care errors. The Speak Up™ program (explained in greater detail in Chapter 3) includes brochures, posters, and buttons on a variety of patient safety topics.

With funding from The California Endowment, The Joint Commission launched the *Hospitals, Language, and Culture* (HLC) study in 2005. Visiting 60 hospitals across the country, researchers gathered qualitative information about the types of programs and activities hospitals are using to provide culturally and linguistically appropriate care. Interviews conducted with administrative and clinical staffs, as well as previsit questionnaires, focused on the areas of leadership, quality improvement and data use, workforce, patient safety and provision of care, language services, and community engagement. So far, the HLC group has published two research reports—

Exploring Cultural and Linguistic Services in the Nation's Hospitals and *One Size Does Not Fit All: Meeting the Health Care Needs of Diverse Populations*—describing the challenges faced by hospitals as they try to serve patients from many disparate cultures and making recommendations for ways of dealing with these challenges.*

Government Efforts

Legislators and government agencies at both the national and state levels have been working to highlight the need for better patient-centered communication and to push for meeting the needs of the diverse populations the health care field serves.

Federal Initiatives

The Minority Health Improvement and Health Disparity Elimination Act (S. 1576), introduced to Congress in June 2007, would amend the Public Health Service Act. Among the actions to be taken, it would require the Secretary of Health & Human Services to support demonstration projects designed to improve the health and health care of minority groups through improved access to health care, health literacy services and education, patient navigators, primary prevention activities, and health promotion and disease prevention activities. The secretary would also be responsible for ensuring data collection in federally supported or conducted health programs regarding race, ethnicity, geographic location, socioeconomic position, primary language, and (when possible) health literacy.[46]

The National Health Literacy Act of 2007 (S. 2424), another amendment to the Public Health Service Act, would require the director of the AHRQ to establish a health literacy implementation center to facilitate solutions to low health literacy. The center would have several responsibilities, as follows:

---

* Both of these reports are available as free downloads at The Joint Commission's Web site. "Exploring Cultural and Linguistic Services in the Nation's Hospitals: A Report of Findings" can be found at http://www.jointcommission.org/PatientSafety/HLC/Exploring_cultutral_and_linguistic_services_in_the_nations_hospital.htm. "One Size Fits All: Meeting the Health Care Needs of a Diverse Population" can be found at http://www.jointcommission.org/PatientSafety/HLC/one_size_meeting_need_of_diverse_populations.htm.

Table 1-3. Culturally and Linguistically Appropriate Services (CLAS) Standards

Culturally Competent Care

Standard 1	Health care organizations should ensure that patients/consumers receive from all staff members effective, understandable, and respectful care that is provided in a manner compatible with their cultural health beliefs and practices and preferred language.
Standard 2	Health care organizations should implement strategies to recruit, retain, and promote at all levels of the organization a diverse staff and leadership that are representative of the demographic characteristics of the service area.
Standard 3	Health care organizations should ensure that staff at all levels and across all disciplines receive ongoing education and training in culturally and linguistically appropriate service delivery.

Language Access Services

Standard 4	Health care organizations must offer and provide language assistance services, including bilingual staff and interpreter services, at no cost to each patient/consumer with limited English proficiency at all points of contact, in a timely manner during all hours of operation.
Standard 5	Health care organizations must provide to patients/consumers in their preferred language both verbal offers and written notices informing them of their right to receive language assistance services.
Standard 6	Health care organizations must ensure the competence of language assistance provided to limited-English-proficient patients/consumers by interpreters and bilingual staff. Family and friends should not be used to provide interpretation services (except on request by the patient/consumer).
Standard 7	Health care organizations must make available easily understood patient-related materials and post signage in the languages of the commonly encountered groups and/or groups represented in the service area.

Organizational Supports for Cultural Competence

Standard 8	Health care organizations should develop, implement, and promote a written strategic plan that outlines clear goals, policies, operational plans, and management accountability/oversight mechanisms to provide culturally and linguistically appropriate services.
Standard 9	Health care organizations should conduct initial and ongoing organizational self-assessments of CLAS–related activities and are encouraged to integrate cultural and linguistic competence-related measures into their internal audits, performance improvement programs, patient satisfaction assessments, and outcomes-based evaluations.
Standard 10	Health care organizations should ensure that data on the individual patient's/consumer's race, ethnicity, and spoken and written language are collected in health records, integrated into the organization's management information systems, and periodically updated.
Standard 11	Health care organizations should maintain a current demographic, cultural, and epidemiological profile of the community, as well as a needs assessment to accurately plan for and implement services that respond to the cultural and linguistic characteristics of the service area.
Standard 12	Health care organizations should develop participatory, collaborative partnerships with communities and utilize a variety of formal and informal mechanisms to facilitate community and patient/consumer involvement in designing and implementing CLAS–related activities.
Standard 13	Health care organizations should ensure that conflict and grievance resolution processes are culturally and linguistically sensitive and capable of identifying, preventing, and resolving cross-cultural conflicts or complaints by patients/consumers.
Standard 14	Health care organizations are encouraged to regularly make available to the public information about their progress and successful innovations in implementing the CLAS standards and to provide public notice in their communities about the availability of this information.

Source: Office of Minority Health: *National Standards on Culturally and Linguistically Appropriate Standards (CLAS)*. U.S. Department of Health & Human Services. http://www.omhrc.gov/templates/browse.aspx?lvl=2&lvlID=15 (last modified Apr. 12, 2007; accessed Jul. 8, 2008).

➤ To make health literacy resources available to researchers, health care providers, and the public

➤ To sponsor demonstration and evaluation projects

➤ To develop health literacy interventions and tools

➤ To identify and fill research gaps relating to health literacy that are directly applicable to quality improvement

➤ To assist federal agencies in establishing specific objectives and strategies for eliminating low literacy and in monitoring programs

➤ To form partnerships to promote the adoption of literacy interventions and tools

➤ To work with the U.S. Department of Health & Human Services (HHS) and the Department of Education to facilitate coordination of health literacy activities within those agencies

Both of these acts are currently being reviewed in committees.

The HHS comprises many agencies that explore the topic of health literacy on an ongoing basis, disseminate information on the problem of low literacy, and support the development of methods and tools to address it. For example, the AHRQ and the Robert Wood Johnson Foundation funded a project by Emory University to develop health literacy tools for pharmacy staff. One tool is an assessment to help staff determine how well they serve patients with low health literacy, and the other is a training program for improving communication between staff and all patients.[47]

Recognizing that a person's ability to understand and accept information is influenced by his or her language and cultural background, the HHS's Office of Minority Health established Culturally and Linguistically Appropriate Services (CLAS) standards in 2001. Directed at health care organizations and individual providers to help them make their services more accessible to all populations, the 14 standards (*see* Table 1-3, page 11) are divided into three categories: culturally competent care, language access services, and organizational supports for cultural competence. The standards dealing with language services are current federal requirements.

Building on earlier initiatives (Healthy People and Healthy People 2000), Health People 2010 is a set of health objectives for the United States to achieve during the first decade of the millennium. Sponsored by the HHS's Office of Disease Prevention and Health Promotion (ODPHP), the program's goals are to increase the quality and length of healthy lives and to eliminate health disparities. To achieve these goals, scientists from the private and public sectors worked together to develop 28 focus areas that identify public health priorities and measurable objectives. For the first time in the Healthy People projects, health communication is included as a focus area, and one of the six objectives of this area is improving health literacy. To help identify appropriate actions for improvement, the ODPHP has published a set of action plans. The strategies included in these plans are intended to focus the attention of researchers, educators, health care providers, and policymakers on raising awareness of the problem, generating new information, motivating funding and the development of innovative policies, promoting monitoring, and encouraging the development of interventions.[48]

Some agencies are trying to improve the readability and usefulness of the information they provide to the public. The National Institute on Aging (NIA) and the National Library of Medicine—both part of the National Institutes of Health (NIH)—have developed the NIHSeniorHealth Web site (http://nihseniorhealth.gov), which is designed specifically to give older adults easy access to authoritative and current health information. Pages feature large print; short, easy-to-read sections; simple navigation; and a "talking" function that reads the text aloud. There is a tool kit to help educators train seniors to use both NIHSeniorHealth and MedlinePlus, another source of health-related information. The NIA also offers free booklets to teach people with low literacy about Alzheimer's disease and memory loss.

State Initiatives

Several states have been working on ways to make care and information more accessible and understandable for all patient populations. For example, representatives from public health agencies, professional associations, health care organizations, insurers, and other stakeholders participate in the Minnesota Alliance for Patient Safety, which develops and disseminates best practices pertaining to patient safety, including health literacy (*see* Chapter 4).

The California Health Literacy program was created because many programs across the state were duplicating efforts, because health literacy was not always addressed effectively by existing health and literacy efforts, and because research was needed to raise the level of awareness of health literacy. The program's four main projects are as follows: (1) partnering with major health care organizations to make health literacy a high priority; (2) establishing an online health literacy resource center that gives everyone access to reliable, understandable Web-based health information; (3) helping to develop measurable health literacy quality standards for Medi-Cal managed-care participants with limited literacy skills; and (4) developing and leading a campaign to raise the awareness of health care professionals and patients about health literacy.

North Carolina's Institute of Medicine, Department of Health & Human Services, and Area Health Education Centers collaborated to form a health literacy task force in 2006, which brought together health care organization and practitioners, state medical associations, patient and consumer advocacy groups, and other stakeholders. The task force developed a list of 14 recommended actions to help serve populations with low health literacy more effectively. These recommendations required the cooperation of all stakeholders and included actions such as having the state Medicaid program pilot test reimbursement models in which providers teach patients self-management, getting malpractice carriers to incorporate information on health literacy into risk management seminars, and encouraging the state's pharmacy board to set requirements for prescription labels and information to make them more understandable for patients with low health literacy.[49]

Pennsylvania established an Interagency Coordinating Council (ICC) in 1996 to improve the delivery and outcomes of basic skills services provided by key state agencies. Recognizing the large number of senior citizens in the state, the ICC sponsored a symposium in 2001 to raise awareness about health literacy among health professionals and key stakeholders, with an emphasis on the issues of aging and health literacy.[50]

Many states—including Georgia, North Carolina, Massachusetts, and Virginia—are endeavoring to make health literacy part of their adult education and English as a Second Language (ESL) courses. For example, Massachusetts has developed Student Health Teams composed of adult learners, teachers, health care professionals, and community health organizations. In a collaborative atmosphere that focuses on peer training and group learning, the teams conduct activities such as finding health information, making and distributing brochures, holding health fairs, and setting up medical screening services.[50] North Carolina's "Expecting the Best" program teaches adults in ESL classes about health and wellness. The curriculum addresses practical skills such as navigating the health care system, making and participating in medical appointments, adhering to treatment plans, and practicing self-care and wellness behaviors.[49]

Actions of Health Care–Related Associations and Groups

Many professional associations and quality organizations have begun focusing on health literacy in their policies and activities. Some concentrate on changing care delivery and communication processes to accommodate the needs of populations with low health literacy; others look at ways of simplifying their own and others' educational materials. Still others work toward improving professional standards and practices.

American Medical Association

The AMA's Code of Medical Ethics states that patients have the right to receive information from their physicians, which involves both the physician giving appropriate information and the patient being able to understand and use it to make decisions.[51] In 1998 the AMA adopted a policy stating that limited patient literacy affects medical diagnosis and treatment. The AMA Foundation has since been working to raise awareness of health literacy through patient safety monographs and partnerships, and in 2003 and 2005, it conducted Health Literacy Train-the-Trainer programs to teach teams how to set up health literacy efforts in their own organizations. The foundation also has tool kits, patient safety tip cards, and a health literacy video/DVD that can be used in a variety of health care settings.

The AMA's Ethical Force Program™ was established in 1997 to advance ethical behavior throughout the health care system. This collaborative research program published a 2006 consensus report on improving communication, which noted that organizations need to consider the health literacy level of their current and potential populations when developing strategies for clear, patient-centered communication. The report also described the three factors that providers must understand to communicate effectively: the audience's culture, language, and health literacy skills.[43]

Partnership for Clear Health Communication (PCHC)

Founded in 2002, PCHC is a nonprofit organization with active members from across the country, including health care organizations, patient advocacy and literacy groups, medical societies, public libraries, universities, and state and local health departments. The organization has the following four main objectives:

1. To expand awareness and educate patients and providers about low health literacy

2. To develop and apply practical strategies to improve patient-provider communication and motivate the health care system to adopt them

3. To advocate for more support of health literacy policy and funding

4. To conduct research to define the health literacy issue and evaluate possible solutions

Ask Me 3™ (*see* Chapter 3), a tool launched in 2003 to help patients understand their diagnoses and follow physician instructions, was PCHC's first solution-based initiative.

Pfizer Health Literacy Initiative

This multidisciplinary program, headed by the company's Public Health Group, was established in 2003 to help patients achieve better outcomes by improving their understanding of health information. Efforts to raise awareness and to encourage more education among providers have included holding a national health literacy conference, forming a partnership with the AMA Foundation, supporting the National Health Council Health Literacy Training program, and providing grants for research. The Pfizer Clear Health Communication Initiative provides facts about health literacy challenges and suggestions for overcoming them for public policymakers and researchers, physicians and other providers, public health professionals, and the media. Its Web site (http://www.pfizerhealthliteracy.com/) has links for tools such as Ask Me 3 and the Newest Vital Sign (for health literacy assessment), as well as the initiative's own set of principles for clear communication with patients.

Other Organizations

Professional associations and national organizations are working to make health literacy a priority in the health care field. For instance, the ACP Foundation established a Patient Literacy Program Focus Policy in late 2003. This policy directs work by the Health Literacy Solutions Program for projects such as promoting informed consent, reducing medical errors, improving health care quality and outcomes, and reducing cultural and language barriers that impede health literacy. The aim is to solve problems created by the prevalence of low health literacy across the country and address these problems from a patient perspective.

Many groups are trying to build provider understanding of the need and ways to counteract low health literacy. For example, in May 2008, the Institute for Healthcare Improvement introduced a Web&ACTION program titled Health Literacy: New Methods for Patient Education and Self-Management Support. It comprised intensive, Web-based learning sessions led by experts in the field, followed by Action Periods during which participants applied their knowledge to specific, detailed assignments in their own organizations. Designed for nurses, physicians, educators, risk managers, case managers, allied health professionals, and others, the goal of the program was threefold:

1. To help participants understand the link between health literacy, quality of care, patient safety, chronic

disease management, health disparities, and patient-centered care

2. To show participants how to evaluate their current patient education materials and processes for improvement opportunities

3. To identify, test, and assess tools and techniques for supporting health care teams in helping patients and families understand medical instructions and information

Both public and private entities are investigating ways of improving both general information that is made available to the public and specific instructions that are given to patients. The U.S. Food and Drug Administration, the American Pharmaceutical Association, the American Society of Health-System Pharmacists, and the National Association of Boards of Pharmacy are directing attention to the quality of drug labels and of educational handouts that are distributed to patients when they receive medications. All of these organizations agree that for the information to be useful, patients must be able to read and understand it before they can act on it.[52]

Many people have trouble finding sources that can provide health information in a specific language. The American Cancer Society's National Cancer Information Center provides information to the public via e-mail or a telephone hotline. Specialists who answer queries speak English and Spanish, and a translation service is available for callers/writers who speak other languages. The Web site (http://www.cancer.org) also has information on wellness-promoting screening and behaviors available in a host of different languages.

Programs Developed by Literacy and Patient Advocates and Others

Entities that try to promote better health literacy through education range from community groups to national organizations, and they focus on everything from specific conditions to general education to consumer information.

On a local level, the AIDS Community Research Initiative of America (ACRIA) has established a comprehensive HIV health literacy program that includes a variety of services. For example, the organization conducts group HIV health literacy workshops and individual health literacy counseling sessions (in English or Spanish) in cooperation with neighborhood-based AIDS service organizations in the New York metropolitan region. ACRIA also has several health literacy publications available on its Web site (http://www.acria.org) and offers a four-day health literacy education and skills-building training program for staff in community-based organizations that provide services to people with HIV.

Incorporating health literacy into adult basic education, secondary education, and ESL classes is the goal of organizations such as the Comprehensive Adult Student Assessment System. This nonprofit organization partners with a national consortium of state and local agencies to provide competency and assessment systems, as well as high school credentialing options through its National External Diploma Program. In this program, students are first assessed for reading, writing, and numeracy skills and interviewed for information on their life experience. They are then given real-life tasks to perform so they can demonstrate competency in areas that include health literacy, writing, speaking, math, problem solving, reading, and critical thinking.

Health literacy advocates and other stakeholders emphasize the importance of introducing health concepts in the schoolroom as early as possible. They believe that offering such education can promote positive health behaviors that will stay with children into adulthood and expose children to health-related tasks that will help them build skills through participation.[53] The need for such education is supported by a 2007 UNICEF report stating that although 90% of U.S. babies are born healthy, the United States has the lowest rating for overall child health and safety out of 21 industrialized countries.[54]

The Joint Committee on National Health Education Standards developed national standards for health education to promote overall health literacy and give state and local schools a framework for developing

Table 1-4. National Health Education Standards	
Standard 1	Students will comprehend concepts related to health promotion and disease prevention to enhance health.
Standard 2	Students will analyze the influence of family, peers, culture, media, technology, and other factors on health behaviors.
Standard 3	Students will demonstrate the ability to access valid information, products, and services to enhance health.
Standard 4	Students will demonstrate the ability to use interpersonal communication skills to enhance health and avoid or reduce health risks.
Standard 5	Students will demonstrate the ability to use decision-making skills to enhance health.
Standard 6	Students will demonstrate the ability to use goal-setting skills to enhance health.
Standard 7	Students will demonstrate the ability to practice health-enhancing behaviors and avoid or reduce health risks.
Standard 8	Students will demonstrate the ability to advocate for personal, family, and community health.

Source: Joint Committee on National Health Education Standards: *National Health Education Standards: Achieving Excellence,* 2nd ed. American Cancer Society, 2007. http://www.cdc.gov/HealthyYouth/SHER/standards/index.htm (accessed Feb. 15, 2009).

health curricula. Children and teens develop their health literacy and advocacy skills by contributing to a class resource file of health information.[8] Each of the eight standards (*see* Table 1-4, page 16) has applicable performance indicators, which are divided by grade level: K–2, 3–5, 6–8, and 9–12.

Many people do not know where to look for health information. Even those with higher levels of health and computer literacy can be stymied by Web sites that are difficult to navigate, that present facts using confusing medical jargon, and that may be unreliable. Low-income and low-literate individuals may not have online access or the necessary skills to gather and interpret information. Part of the National Network of Libraries of Medicine's mission is to improve public access to the information necessary to make informed health decisions, and libraries have been urged to reach out to low-literate groups in their communities. The Community Outreach Information Network (COIN) in Richmond, Virginia, comprises four consumer health information centers and has holdings in multiple languages and formats. COIN provides access to print materials and the Internet and offers face-to-face and telephone reference assistance, as well as a virtual reference service that allows users to interact electronically with a medical librarian. A COIN Web site

(http://www.library.vcu.edu/coin) posts information about local resources and provides quick links to reliable health information in English and Spanish. A 2006 survey showed that many users of the COIN centers were referred by physicians or nurses.[55]

Access to language services is also an important issue for improving health literacy among LEP populations. A national coalition of health care organizations, professional associations, advocacy groups, and interpreter and accrediting organizations has created a theoretical guide for addressing language access issues in health care. Coordinated by the National Health Law Program and supported by The California Endowment, the Language Access in Health Statement of Principles lists 11 basic tenets covering the topics of access to and funding of services, staff training, assessment of services, and accountability for providing services. The suggestions and rationales incorporated in these principles are directed toward providers; public health agencies; insurers; and federal, state, and local policymakers.[56]

The Need for Private–Public Cooperation

Practitioners and health care organizations alone cannot improve the health literacy of their patient populations. In *Health Literacy: A Prescription to End Confusion,* the IOM made several recommendations to combat limited health literacy, including expanding health literacy research; creating new measures for health literacy, including communication and awareness of literacy issues in the curricula for health care professionals; identifying methods for reducing the effects of poor health literacy; following applicable standards from accrediting bodies; and implementing national health education standards.[2] These recommendations would necessitate collaboration among health care organizations, government agencies and policymakers, universities, professional associations, accrediting entities, patient advocacy groups, and many others. Given the shortage of nurses and other health professionals available to provide patient education, stakeholders such as the public health system, the public education system, and the media will need to accept responsibility for providing health-related materials that are understandable to people at all literacy levels and thus will help to improve the nation's health literacy level.[57]

In a 2005 commentary on public health literacy, the AMA acknowledged that the push to improve health literacy was gaining momentum and recommended that all disciplines share expertise to make the issue a public health priority. According to the authors, "We need to reach out and learn from other fields in our society that reach the public such as the adult education community, communications sectors, and marketing specialists."[51]

Adult education is the most obvious place to begin. The link between health literacy and general literacy means that adult education programs and ESL classes are the perfect places to build skills related to both. Instructors can be flexible in choosing what materials they use, and their teaching methods are designed specifically for adult learners, many of whom are at high risk for limited health literacy. Adult learners can be motivated to apply their growing language and numeracy skills to health-related activities such as reading nutritional labels on food packages, understanding appointment reminders, using directories of health care providers, filling out applications from health care plans, and interpreting standard informed consent forms. Also, because all students tend to be at the same literacy level, they can feel more comfortable admitting that they do

not understand something, asking for help, and sharing their frustrations and successes with other students than they would in other settings.[42,58]

Many suggestions have been made about how stakeholders from every facet of the health care system can help to alleviate the problems of poor health literacy. The following are a few of these recommendations:

Recommendations

➤ Policymakers, professional organizations, government agencies, and the health care industry as a whole should work together to standardize and possibly regulate the content and dissemination of patient information.[59]

➤ Health systems should be simplified so they require patients to complete fewer tasks.[59]

➤ Performance measures of patient experience should adequately capture the experiences of patients with limited health literacy.[60]

➤ Health care organizations and systems should receive financial rewards for investing in programs to improve health literacy and in technology that supports patient education and self-care.[60]

➤ The federal government could encourage health literacy by creating centers of excellence to promote the study of health literacy and the adoption of best practices to improve it.[38]

➤ Health literacy skills should become a basic component of federally supported health professions' education and training programs.[38]

How does all of this affect what you are doing in your organization or practice? Any health care professional in any setting may deal with patients who have low health literacy. As communities become increasingly more diverse, the number of older adults increase, and the high school drop-out rate remains high, the odds are good that you need to look at your patient population more closely and determine what its health literacy needs are so you can help your patients improve their overall health and avoid adverse events. Chapter 2 contains suggestions for evaluating your patients and collecting and tracking data pertaining to health literacy.

References

1. Agency for Healthcare Research and Quality: Only about 1 in 10 adult Americans have all the skills needed to manage their health. *AHRQ News and Numbers,* May 14, 2008. http://www.ahrq.gov/news/nn/nn051408.htm (accessed Dec. 30, 2008).
2. Nielsen-Bohlman L.N., Panzer A.M., Kindig D.A. (eds.): *Health Literacy: A Prescription to End Confusion.* Washington, DC: National Academies Press, 2004.
3. Zarcadoolas C., Pleasant A., Greer D.S.: Understanding health literacy: An expanded model. *Health Promot Int* 20(2):195–203, 2005.
4. Nutbeam D.: Health literacy as a public health goal: A challenge for contemporary health education and communication strategies into the 21st century. *Health Promot Int* 15(3):259–267, 2000.
5. Parker R.M., et al.: The Test of Functional Health Literacy in Adults: A new instrument for measuring patients' literacy skills. *J Gen Intern Med* 10:537–541, 1995.
6. Coles M.E., Coleman S., Heimberg R.G.: Addressing patient needs: The role of mental health literacy. *Am J Psychiatry* 163:399, Mar. 2008.
7. Renkert S., Nutbeam D.: Opportunities to improve maternal health literacy through antenatal education: An exploratory study. *Health Promot Int* 16(4):381–388, 2001.
8. Brey R.A., Clark S.E., Wantz M.S.: Enhancing health literacy through accessing health information, products, and services: An exercise for children and adolescents. *J Sch Health* 77:640–644, Nov. 2007.
9. Foubister V.: Health literacy—A quality and patient safety imperative. *Quality Matters: Health Literacy* 21, The Commonwealth Fund, Nov.–Dec. 2006. http://www.commonwealthfund.org/publications/publications_show.htm?doc_id=424780 (accessed Dec. 30, 2008).
10. Kutner M., et al.: *The Health Literacy of America's Adults: Results from the 2003 National Assessment of Adult Literacy.* (NCES 2006-483). Washington, DC: U.S. Department of Education, National Center for Education Statistics, 2006.
11. Kirsch I., et al.: *Adult Literacy in America: The First Look at the Results of the National Adult Literacy Survey (NALS).* Washington, DC: U.S. Department of Education, 1993.
12. Brown H., et al.: *Literacy of Older Adults in America: Results from the National Adult Literacy Survey.* Washington, DC: U.S. Department of Education, 1996.
13. Sum A., Kirsch I., Taggart R.: *The Twin Challenges of Mediocrity and Inequality: Literacy in the U.S. from an International Perspective.* Princeton, N.J.: Educational Testing Service, Center for Global Assessment, 2002.
14. Tuijnman A.: *Benchmarking Adult Literacy in America: An International Comparative Study.* Washington, DC: U.S. Department of Education, 2000.
15. Rudd R., Kirsch I., Yamamoto K.: *Literacy and Health in America.* Princeton, NJ: Educational Testing Service, Center for Global Assessment, 2004.
16. Kirsch I., Braun H., Yamamoto K.: *America's Perfect Storm: Three Forces Changing Our Nation's Future.* Princeton, NJ: Educational Testing Service, 2007.
17. Corbeil J-P.: *The Canadian Component of the 2003 International Adult Literacy and Skills Survey (IALSS): The Situation of Official Language Minorities.* Ottawa: Minister of Industry, 2006.
18. Statistics Canada: International Adult Literacy and Skills Survey. *The Daily,* Nov. 9, 2005. http://www.statcan.gc.ca/daily-quotidien/051109/dq051109a-eng. htm (accessed Dec. 30, 2008).
19. The California Health Literacy Initiative: *Low Literacy, High Risk: The Hidden Challenge Facing Health Care in California.* Oct. 2003. http://cahealthliteracy.org/pdffiles/healthliteracylongreport012704_3.pdf (accessed Dec. 30, 2008).
20. American Cancer Society: *Worsening Health Trends Among Least Educated.* May 14, 2008. http://www.cancer.org/docroot/NWS/content/NWS_1_1x_Worsening_Health_Trends_Among_Least_Educated.asp (accessed Dec. 30, 2008).
21. The Joint Commission: *"What Did the Doctor Say?" Improving Health Literacy to Protect Patient Safety* (white paper). Oakbrook Terrace, IL: 2007.
22. Baker D.W., et al.: Functional health literacy and the risk of hospital admission among Medicare managed care enrollees. *Am J Public Health* 92(8):1278–1283, 2002.
23. Agency for Healthcare Research and Quality: *Literacy and Health Outcomes.* Evidence Report/Technology Assessment Number 87. AHRQ Publication No. 04-E007-2. Rockville, MD: U.S. Department of Health & Human Services, Jan. 2004.
24. Cho Y.I., et al.: Effects of health literacy on health status and health service utilization amongst the elderly. *Soc Sci Med* 66:1809–1816, 2008.
25. Baker D.W., et al.: Health literacy and mortality among elderly persons. *Arch Intern Med* 167:1503–1509, Jul. 23, 2007.
26. Valenti W.M.: Health literacy, HIV, and outcomes. *AIDS Read* 17:124, Mar. 1, 2007.
27. Lindau S.T., Basu A., Leitsch S.A.: Health literacy as a predictor of follow-up after an abnormal Pap smear: A prospective study. *J Gen Intern Med* 21:829–834, 2006.
28. Baker D.W.: Reading between the lines: Deciphering the connection between literacy and health [editorial]. *J Gen Intern Med* 14:315–317, May 1999.
29. Weiss B.D.: Epidemiology of low health literacy. In Schwartzberg J.G., VanGeest J.B., Wang C.C. (eds.): *Understanding Health Literacy: Implications for Medicine and Public Health.* Chicago: American Medical Association, 2005, pp. 17–39.
30. Riley J.B., Cloonan P., Norton C.: Low health literacy: A challenge to critical care. *Crit Care Nurs Q* 29(2):174–178, 2006.
31. Miller D.P. Jr., et al.: The effect of health literacy on knowledge and receipt of colorectal cancer screening: A survey study. *BMC Fam Pract* 8, Mar. 30, 2007. http://www.biomedcentral.com/1471-2296/8/16 (accessed Dec. 30, 2008).
32. Davis T.C., et al.: The role of inadequate health literacy skills in colorectal cancer screening. *Cancer Invest* 19(2):193–200, 2001.
33. Howard D.H., Gazmararian J., Parker R.M.: The impact of low health literacy on the medical costs of Medicare managed care enrollees. *Am J Med* 118(4):371–377, 2005.
34. Baker D.W., et al.: Health literacy and the risk of hospital admission. *J Gen Intern Med* 13:791–798, 1998.
35. Center on an Aging Society, Georgetown University: *Low Health Literacy Skills Increase Annual Health Care Expenditures by $73 Billion.* http://hpi.georgetown.edu/agingsociety/pubhtml/healthlit.html (acessed Dec. 30, 2008).
36. Agency for Healthcare Research and Quality: Problems with English help block many Hispanics from medical care. *AHRQ News and Numbers,* Mar. 26, 2008. http://www.ahrq.gov/news/nn/nn032608.htm (accessed Dec. 30, 2008).
37. Pippins J.R., Alegria M., Haas J.S.: Association between language proficiency and the quality of primary care among a national sample of insured Latinos. *Med Care* 45:1020–1025, Nov. 2007.
38. Vernon J.A., et al.: *Low Health Literacy: Implications for National Health Policy.* http://www.npsf.org/askme3/pdfs/Case_Report_10_07.pdf (accessed Aug. 30, 2008).
39. Williams M.V., et al.: Inadequate functional health literacy among patients at two public hospitals. *JAMA* 274:1677–1682, 1995.
40. Weiss B.D., Palmer R.: Relationship between health care costs and very low literacy skills in a medically needy and indigent Medicaid population. *J Am Board Fam Pract* 17:44–47, 2004.
41. Partnership for Clear Health Communication: *What Is Health Literacy?* http://www.npsf.org/pchc/health-literacy.php (accessed Dec. 30, 2008).
42. Sherow S.: Health literacy: Issues with implications for adult education. *Pennsylvania ABLE Administrators Fieldnotes.* Commonwealth of Pennsylvania, 2003. http://www.able.state.pa.us/able/lib/able/fieldnotes03/fn03healthlit.pdf (accessed Dec. 30, 2008).

43. American Medical Association: *Improving Communication—Improving Care: An Ethical Force Program*™ *Consensus Report.* Chicago: American Medical Association, 2006.

44. Schyve P.M.: Language differences as a barrier to quality and safety in health care: The Joint Commission perspective. *J Gen Intern Med* 22(suppl. 2):360–361, 2007.

45. Murphy-Knoll L.: Low health literacy puts patients at risk: The Joint Commission proposes solutions to national problem. *J Nurs Care Qual* 22:205–209, Jul.–Sep. 2007.

46. GovTrack.us: *S. 1576: Minority Health Improvement and Health Disparity Elimination Act.* Updated Jun. 15, 2008. http://www.govtrack.us/congress/bill.xpd?bill=s110-1576&tab=summary (accessed Dec. 30, 2008).

47. Agency for Healthcare Research and Quality: *Press Release: New AHRQ Tools Help Pharmacies Better Serve Patients with Limited Health Literacy.* Oct. 30, 2007. http://www.ahrq.gov/news/press/pr2007/pharmtoolpr.htm (accessed Dec. 30, 2008).

48. Office of Disease Prevention and Health Promotion, U.S. Department of Health & Human Services: *Healthy People 2010.* http://www.healthypeople.gov (accessed Dec. 30, 2008).

49. Holmes M., et al.: Addressing health literacy through improved patient-practitioner communication. *N C Med J* 68:319–326, Sep.–Oct. 2007.

50. Hohn M.D.: Literacy, health, and health literacy: State policy considerations. *Focus on Basics: Connecting Research and Practice* 5, Feb. 2002. http://www.ncsall.net/?id=243 (accessed Dec. 30, 2008).

51. Nelson J.C., Schwartzberg J.G., Vergara K.C.: The public's and the patient's right to know: AMA commentary on "Public Health in America: An Ethical Imperative." *Am J Prev Med* 28(3):325–326, 2005.

52. Davis T.C., et al.: Literacy and misunderstanding prescription drug labels. *Ann Intern Med* 145:887–894, Dec. 19, 2006.

53. Amercian Cancer Society, American Diabetes Association, American Heart Association: *Health Education in Schools—The Importance of Establishing Healthy Behaviors in Our Nation's Youth.* Sep. 3, 2008. http://www.ncaahperd.org/pdf/health.pdf (accessed Dec. 30, 2008).

54. United Nations Children's Fund: *Child Poverty in Perspective: An Overview of Child Well-Being in Rich Countries.* 2007. http://www.unicef.org/media/files/ChildPovertyReport.pdf (accessed Dec. 30, 2008).

55. Kennedy M.G., Kiken L., Shipman J.P.: Addressing underutilization of consumer health information resource centers: A formative study. *J Med Libr Assoc* 96:42–49, Jan. 2008.

56. Martinez E.L., Hitov S., Youdelman M.: *Language Access in Health Care Statement of Principles: Explanatory Guide.* National Health Law Program. Oct. 2006. http://www.hablamosjuntos.org/newsletters/2006/October/pdf/LanguageAccessExplanatoryGuide_2006_Martinez.pdf (accessed Dec. 30, 2008).

57. Rao P.R.: Health literacy: The cornerstone of patient safety. *ASHA Leader* 12:8–9, 20, May 8, 2007.

58. Diehl S.J.: Incorporating health literacy into adult basic education: From life skills to life saving. *N C Med J* 68:336–339, Sep.–Oct. 2007.

59. Parker R.M., Wolf M.S., Kirsch I.: Preparing for an epidemic of limited health literacy: Weathering the perfect storm. *J Gen Intern Med* 23:1273–1276, Aug. 2008.

60. Paasche-Orlow M.K., et al.: How health care systems can begin to address the challenge of limited literacy. *J Gen Intern Med* 21:884–887, 2006.

CHAPTER 2

ASSESSING HEALTH LITERACY

Before you can address your patient population's health literacy needs, you must know what those needs are. Although many experts advocate a "universal precautions" approach—meaning that all discussions and materials are simple enough for everyone to understand, regardless of literacy level—some patient encounters will demand special consideration and planning. Patients' command of English or cultural backgrounds, physical or mental disabilities, and so on will influence your communication style and the types of educational materials you use. In this chapter, we will look at various ways of evaluating individual patients and populations for information that can help you tailor your health literacy efforts.

Identifying High-Risk and Vulnerable Populations

According to the 2003 National Assessment of Adult Literacy (NAAL), certain demographic characteristics correlate with specific levels of health literacy,[1] as follows:

➤ Starting with adults who had graduated from high school or obtained a general equivalency diploma (GED), average health literacy increased with each consecutive level of education. About 49% of those who had never attended or did not complete high school had below basic health literacy, compared with 15% of high school graduates and 3% of college graduates.

➤ People living below the poverty level exhibited lower health literacy levels than those with higher incomes.

➤ Adults age 65 and older had lower average health literacy than younger people.

➤ Adults whose first language was English had higher health literacy levels than those who had never learned English or who spoke it as a second language.

➤ White and Asian/Pacific Islander adults had higher average health literacy than black, Hispanic, Native American/Alaska Native, and multiracial adults. Hispanic adults had the lowest average health literacy of any racial or ethnic group.

Although the survey's results were much more extensive, these facts show that the risk for poor health literacy is greatly affected by education, income, age, English proficiency, and race and cultural background.

Education and Income

Many elements influence a person's level of health literacy. The most obvious involves the ability to read, write, and understand the text and numbers used to present information. Studies have shown a correlation between less education and earlier mortality, usually due to a greater tendency toward risky health behaviors (*see* Chapter 1).[2] People with lower levels of education or general literacy are also at a disadvantage in communicating with health care professionals. They may have limited vocabularies and not be able to express symptoms clearly; for example, they may be unable to distinguish between *tingling, stinging, aching,* or *throbbing* when asked to describe their pain. Although terms such as *hyperpyrexia* or *reticuloendothelial system* can be difficult for anyone to decipher, those with low literacy may not even comprehend words such as *tumor, lesion,* or *growth,*[3] particularly when they are used interchangeably or in an unfamiliar context.

Education level also generally correlates to occupation and income. People with degrees beyond the high school level tend to have more knowledge-intensive jobs (accountant, lawyer, architect, clinician, educator, computer programmer, corporate manager, and so on), higher functional literacy levels, and higher incomes.[4] Income, in turn, can affect whether someone can afford health insurance, and literacy level can determine whether a low-income individual can figure out how to apply for aid. In the 2003 NAAL, people who received health insurance coverage through their employer, a family member's employer, or the military—or who purchased insurance on their own—had higher health literacy scores than those who received Medicare or Medicaid or had no insurance.[1]

Age

America's baby boomers are aging, and the growing number of senior citizens requires all providers of health care information to consider the special needs of older adults. More than 75% of the current Medicare population has one or more chronic conditions, and in less than 20 years, the care of these conditions will account for 80% of U.S. health care spending.[5]

Varying levels of cognitive ability, sometimes caused or exacerbated by medication, mean that elderly patients often find it difficult to comprehend either written or verbal information regarding their medical conditions or treatment options. Senior citizens may also suffer from physical impairments such as failing eyesight or hearing, which can reduce their ability to understand information, or neurological disorders that affect their speech and language abilities, which can make it impossible for them to communicate with physicians or educators.[6]

Although four out of five Americans age 65 and over scored in the two lowest levels for document literacy in the National Adult Literacy Survey (see Chapter 1), many of them did not believe that they had any trouble with literacy. Although many admitted to receiving help with writing letters, filling out forms, and so on, the survey found that the number of seniors who get help is much lower than the number of those who need it.[7] For example, comparing Medicare supplements, understanding the rules imposed by Medicare and secondary insurers, and finding ways to cut medication costs are

other areas that require patients to be able to seek out and understand information from government sources, insurance companies, and pharmaceutical companies. Many older adults may find it intimidating to try to find the information they need online, and even those who are Internet-savvy may not be able to navigate complex health care–related sites or find information that is presented so they can understand it.

Seniors may be afraid to ask practitioners for clarification for a variety of reasons. Most grew up with the traditional paternalistic mind-set that physicians are always right and should not be questioned or challenged. Even if elderly patients are willing to participate more fully in their care, they may not know what questions to ask. Many are also reluctant to admit they do not understand for fear of being judged incompetent and/or that they are losing their autonomy.

English Proficiency

Low health literacy is particularly prevalent in people who do not speak English or who have limited English proficiency (LEP). According to an American Medical Association report, more than 22 million people in the United States speak English less than "very well," and more than 34 million people were born in another country.[8] Staff members in an urban hospital may hear as many as 80 different languages from their patient population. A great number of immigrants find it almost impossible to communicate. For example, 61% of Vietnamese, 51% of Chinese, and 24% of Filipinos in the United States do not speak any English.[9] In 2000 the most common languages spoken, other than English and Spanish, were Chinese, French, German, Tagalog, Vietnamese, Italian, Korean, Russian, Polish, and Arabic.[10]

Traditionally, health care staff allowed family members or friends to interpret for patients. This practice is now strongly discouraged, but The Joint Commission's *Hospitals, Language, and Culture* (HLC) study found that few organizations had policies that prohibited it.[11] There is no way to tell whether such interpretations are accurate or whether the interpreter has edited information based on his or her own beliefs or level of comprehension. Patients also may not wish to re-lay sensitive information about finances or physical health through someone else, particularly a child. Although in-house interpreter services are becoming more common, many organizations may use bilingual staff that have not been trained or evaluated as medical interpreters. Others may use dial-up services that provide interpreters for different languages over the phone.

The informed consent process is an area where the patient's complete understanding is crucial, yet consent forms are often translated into only a limited number of languages, with Spanish being the most prevalent. Because the process involves more than just a signature, accurate interpretation of both the physician's explanations and the patient's questions is essential for true consent to be given. However, many practitioners still do not see the need for an interpreter if they have a translated form.[11]

Providing educational materials in a needed language can also be problematic. Translation is not a straightforward science, because the same language may have many dialects, and the meaning of a word can change from one dialect to another.

Whether trained interpreters or well-translated materials are used, there is still the question of whether patients are health literate in their own language. As with English-speaking populations, knowledge in this area is determined by level of education, socioeconomic status, cultural background, and so on.

Race and Culture

The wide range of languages heard in many health care organizations comes as no surprise when you consider that during the 1990s the number of foreign-born people in the United States nearly doubled. According to 2008 U.S. Census Bureau estimates, there are approximately 44 million people of Hispanic and Latino descent and 13 million of Asian descent residing in this country, and the numbers keep growing.[12]

Each of these groups has its own set of cultural beliefs and mores. Religion, family dynamics, and values

also inform how patients learn and communicate about health and illness. The following are some aspects of medical care and the patient experience that can be affected by cultural background[13]:

➤ Understanding of a diagnosis
➤ Trust in and compliance with a plan of treatment
➤ Reporting of symptoms
➤ Desire for information
➤ Attitudes toward death and dying
➤ Gender roles
➤ Family participation in care
➤ Decision making

Further, general perceptions of health or of "what is healthy" may also be driven by culture and can have a huge impact on clinical encounters, affecting patient-provider communication, treatment adherence, and so forth.

Depending on the situation, several aspects may come into play at once. For example, some Hispanic men ignore symptoms until the need for medical treatment is urgent; even then, they may downplay the number or degree of symptoms they have experienced because they believe that illness is a sign of weakness and that men should never admit to weakness. People from many areas of the world, including Europeans, Asians, and Native Americans, regularly use complementary treatments such as herbal remedies, acupuncture/acupressure, and traditional Chinese medicine. Some may see the practice of medicine as having a spiritual element rather being merely scientific. Patients may actually be uncomfortable with a physician, nurse, educator, or other professional of a different race, culture, age, or gender. Because of this, they may ignore or misconstrue information, even when it is presented clearly in their preferred language. All of this makes raising health literacy levels challenging.

None of these examples is meant to stereotype individual groups or to imply that everyone from a specific cultural background will react the same way to providers and health information. In fact, there is some evidence that immigrants may begin to take on the attitudes and conditions of their adopted country. One study reported that recent Asian immigrants were less likely than whites to report symptoms of stress, but Asian immigrants who had lived in the United States for 15 years or more reported higher stress levels, suggesting that those who were more acclimated to American culture were either better able or more willing to recognize stress factors.[14]

Misconceptions About Who Is at Risk

Although the groups already described are at higher risk than most for low health literacy, demographics are not the deciding factor in whether a patient understands health information. Many health care professionals find it difficult to believe that their patients may not comprehend explanations of diagnoses or facts given in educational brochures, particularly if those patients speak English, have a college education, and/or are in occupations demanding specialized skills. But appearances can be deceiving. A pharmacy technician who reads at the seventh-grade level or an architect who has had no experience in the health care system aside from yearly wellness checkups may function perfectly well in their daily lives but be mystified by discussions of medical conditions or written instructions for how to prepare for tests or surgery. Urmimala Sarkar, M.D., M.P.H., Assistant Professor, Division of General Internal Medicine at the University of California, San Francisco, explains this "demand-capacity mismatch": "Health systems demand a higher level of literacy than most other areas of people's lives. You can graduate from high school or do quite skilled work and have limited health literacy to the point that it affects your health."

This is particularly relevant for ambulatory patients. Those with chronic diseases such as asthma, diabetes, HIV, and hypertension have to deal with many self-management issues, including the high acuity of their condition, stringent treatment goals, often-complicated medication instructions, and frequent primary care visits. "Ambulatory patients are driving the boat, whereas patients in the hospital are under constant observation, and care is delivered to them," notes Sarkar. "The demand on ambulatory patients, especially chronic disease patients, is much higher because they have to perform all of their self-care actions, and mistakes or gaps in knowledge can take longer to come to [providers'] attention."

Sarkar and a team of researchers learned this first-hand in a nine-month study that was intended to investigate diabetes self-management. In a three-arm trial, diabetes patients who were being actively followed by a primary care physician (at least two visits within the preceding 12 months) and whose condition was not well controlled were randomized to automated phone calls (with a live nurse follow-up), usual care, or group educational sessions. In the first group, patients received weekly automated phone calls on a diabetes self-management topic such as exercise, managing blood sugar, or taking medication regularly. They first listened to a narrative about how a person in a similar life situation overcame difficulties with self-management, then answered some related questions by using the telephone touchpad; for example, if the question was "What was your last blood sugar?" they entered the number. These responses were reviewed by a nurse care manager who called patients whose responses were outside pre-specified parameters.

What these phone calls revealed was that some patients were experiencing health problems that they did not realize required medical attention. For example, a woman with extremely high blood sugar reported during the follow-up call that she thought it was due to the fever she was experiencing with her urinary tract infection; she had not been to her clinic and was receiving no antibiotics. A man who had stopped exercising regularly explained that it was because of an open sore on his foot that caused pain when he walked; he had not reported this problem to his physician. "This study wasn't originally intended to look at patient safety, but we found that people were reporting adverse events," recalls Sarkar. "Patient safety problems in the ambulatory setting happen because providers and health systems do not adequately equip chronic disease patients to perform daily self-management and recognize potentially dangerous symptoms." The researchers identified 111 adverse events and 153 potential adverse events among the 111 participants, 54% of whom were determined to have low health literacy. Although most of the events had several contributing causes, 55% involved poor patient–provider communication, whether with physicians, nurses, or pharmacists.[15]

Circumstances also affect how well people can absorb and use information. A college-educated mother of three who has been up for two consecutive nights with a sick child, or a nurse who is taking high doses of pain medication for a back injury, may usually be health literate, but their immediate situations make it difficult or impossible to make an informed decision. Patients and families who are under extreme stress, such as those in a critical care unit, are particularly vulnerable. They have little or no time to make vital health care decisions about a situation that is already physically and emotionally draining due to the severity of the patient's condition. The patient may be cognitively impaired because of his or her health status or having received pain medications or sedation. Family members or other caregivers who may be put in the position of making decisions for the patient need information about proposed interventions, the equipment and medications being used, and the prognosis, but this information is often difficult to come by.[16] Under these conditions, people often feel confused, angry, and afraid, so that even those with normally high health literacy may not know what to do.

The important thing to remember is that an accurate assessment of a patient's (or family member's) health literacy level cannot be based solely on how that person looks, what language he or she speaks, or how far he or she went in school.

Patient Behaviors That Hide Poor Health Literacy

Because so many people are ashamed to admit that they have limited literacy skills or problems understanding information, you may need to look for certain behaviors and cues that can indicate poor health literacy. For example, when asked to fill out registration or medical history forms, patients may become angry or leave before they complete the form, hand in forms that are incomplete or have many misspelled words, ask for help reading the form (often explaining, "I forgot my glasses"), or ask to fill the form out at home because they are in a hurry or wish to show it to a family member.[17-19]

Patients may frequently miss appointments for physician visits, diagnostic procedures, or referrals to other settings or services. When asked to explain what medications they take, they may only be able to describe the drug's appearance, without knowing the name or what it is for; they may also be unclear on dosing schedules.[17-19] For example, family members often help senior citizens manage their multiple medications by filling pillboxes for a week, with doses divided by day and time (breakfast, lunch, dinner, and bedtime). Nurses and physicians who ask about medications commonly hear responses such as "I take that pink pill for depression," or "I have a white pill that I take three times a day."

Problems with sight or hearing frequently influence how much information someone can extract from a brochure or conversation; unfortunately, many individuals do not want to acknowledge these disabilities, particularly when the onset is gradual. Accusations of "It's too dark in here," or "You're mumbling," generally indicate problems in this area.

Patients who are reluctant to ask questions for any reason, particularly in LEP populations, may simply smile and nod to indicate understanding where none exists. They become adept at reading facial expressions, and when asked a question, they try a nod or headshake first; if you seem confused, they switch to the other. If you ask them an open-ended question that requires a specific answer instead of a yes or no response, they will look at you blankly.

Keep in mind that high-income, well-educated, English-speaking patients may be just as prone to poor health literacy as low-income, poorly educated, LEP patients. The former are far more likely to hide their lack of skills, so being on the lookout for these behaviors can help you identify those who might need extra help.

Discussion Techniques for Spotting Poor Health Literacy

All staff members in your organization or practice should be alert to possible health literacy problems. Informal conversations or questions that are posed as just another part of the assessment or visit can help you judge patients' needs without making them feel embarrassed or defensive.

Questions to Ask

Initial assessment questions might include "How do you prefer to learn?" or "Would you like to receive written materials about what your physician tells you?" to help you identify the best way to present information. For example, if a patient prefers written materials to verbal instructions, either he or she may want to take them home so a friend or family member can explain them, or it may indicate that you need to use visual aids as part of your discussion.

You may choose to use variations of the questions suggested here, depending on the needs of your organization and patients. For example, workers at a university-based vascular surgery center in Tennessee found that they could predict limited and marginal health literacy using the screening questions "How confident are you filling out medical forms by yourself?" and "How often do you have someone (like a family member, friend, of hospital worker) help you read materials?"[20]

Assessing family members' level of health literacy can be done in much the same way as it is for patients. You can pose open-ended questions in informal conversation, ask them to read written health information, and/or use one of the standardized assessment tools discussed later in this chapter. You may wish to introduce the assessment process by explaining that because family members are such an important component of the care experience, you will ask both the patient and family member for information. It may also be helpful to give family members their own set of written materials and/or instructions that duplicates what is given to the patient.[21]

Brown-Bag Medication Reviews

Medication reconciliation can be an ongoing challenge for patients with low health literacy, particularly if they see one or more specialists in addition to their primary care physician and/or if they purchase their medications through several different venues (mail-order versus pharmacy-with-insurance versus discount pharmacy) to get the best prices. In a study of English-speaking patients being treated for hypertension, only 22.7% of patients could name two or more of their medications, and 40.3% could not name any of them.[22]

Conducting a "brown-bag" medication review with patients can help you evaluate their health literacy skills related to drug regimens. Ask patients to bring all of their medications—including prescriptions, over-the-counter remedies, and supplements—to their appointments. Then ask for an explanation of each medication: the name, what it is used for, and when and how often they take it. Observe *how* they answer the questions as well as *what* their responses are. For instance, do they need to see an actual pill before they can identify its purpose? Do they struggle with the pronunciation of the name? Do they have trouble describing their administration schedule even after rereading the package instructions? Can they interpret the warning labels on prescription bottles correctly? All of these indicators can give you clues that should be followed up.

Teach-Back After Education

You can use teach-back (described in detail in Chapter 3) after you have explained a condition or diagnosis, medication choices, a proposed plan of care, or other information to a patient. Rather than asking if the patient has any questions, request that he or she repeat back what you've just said in his or her own words. This will help you assess whether the patient has understood the important points and/or will be able to follow any instructions given. The need to repeat a discussion more than once means that you need to find a way to present your information more clearly and simply.

Standardized Assessment Tools

Many health care organizations choose not to use assessment tools for literacy, usually because of concerns about the time and resources involved or the possibility of patients responding negatively.[23,24] "Testing may be off-putting for many people," explains Terry Davis, Ph.D., Department of Medicine, Louisiana State University Health Sciences Center, Shreveport. "When we administer the REALM [Rapid Estimate of Adult Literacy in Medicine], we don't use the words *test* or *to read,* but people still realize they're being tested." Facilities may instead attempt to make all of their materials and processes easy to understand for all patients. According to Davis, "If you're going to use standardized tests, you should use the aggregate results to get a realistic picture of a general or specific patient population, or if you're using them in individual clinical settings, you need to do something with the information, such as tailoring your communications or patient education or developing special programs for groups you identify."

This is not to say that standardized tests are not useful for certain activities. Baker and colleagues suggest that when patients are being asked to follow complicated treatment regimens, such as those for HIV and other chronic diseases, they should be screened at the start of any instructional program to determine their literacy skills.[25] You may also want to use tests to create a profile of a specific population's skills so you can develop appropriate educational materials or to conduct research (such as testing for correlations between literacy level and other measures such as control of glucose level or blood pressure, compliance with care plans, or use of specific services).

Widely Used Tests

If you choose to screen patients using a standardized method, you should keep a couple of things in mind. No matter which test you use or where you administer it, always approach potential participants with respect and sensitivity so they do not feel as though they are being singled out or judged. Most people will be more willing to join in if you explain simply and honestly why you are conducting the test and if you ask for their help in gathering information.[26] For example, you might try something like "We are writing some new booklets about ways to cope with illness, and we want them to be easy to understand. To do this, we need to know what words our patients find difficult. Would you help me gather information by taking this brief test?" If someone refuses, respect his or her decision and move on.[26]

Also remember that a person may score fairly high on a reading or numeracy test but not necessarily know how to use their skills appropriately. Medical situations demand that patients be able to understand new material and apply it to their existing knowledge so that it can be retained in memory and recalled when needed. The screening tools described here can help you estimate levels of literacy, but they cannot identify specific learning disabilities or the reasons for low levels.

This section looks at the three tests used most frequently in health care settings (all of which have been tested for validity and reliability), as well as some alternative screening methods. The worksheet in Figure 2-1 (page 28) will help you decide which test is best for your purpose and how you will use it. Ordering information for the three main tests is given in the Appendix at the back of this book.

REALM

The REALM is a word recognition test in which you ask patients to read aloud a series of 66 words and terms commonly used in clinical settings (*see* Figure 2-2, page 29). The words are split into three lists and progress from easy, single-syllable items to multisyllable terms that are more difficult to pronounce. You can administer and score the test in two to three minutes. Patients receive one point for each word they say correctly (meaning exactly as it is written—singular versus plural, and so on; and according to dictionary pronunciation).[27]

To make the test even faster to use, a very brief version has been developed. The REALM–Short Form (REALM-SF) uses only seven of the words from the original lists (menopause, antibiotics, exercise, jaundice, rectal, anemia, and behavior). It can be administered in a minute or less.[28]

A version of the REALM is also available for use with teens (Rapid Estimate of Adolescent Literacy in Medicine, or REALM-Teen). As with the test for adults, the one-page tool has 66 words given in increasing order of difficulty; however, these terms are taken from patient education materials for adolescents published by the Academy of Pediatrics. The test sheet is printed on lime green paper. Patients again receive one point for each correctly pronounced word, but the scoring differs from that used in the adult REALM. Here, 0–37 indicates 3rd grade or below, 38–44 is 4th or 5th grade, 45–58 is 6th to 7th grade, 59–62 is 8th to 9th grade, and 63–66 is 10th grade or above.[29]

Test of Functional Health Literacy in Adults

The Test of Functional Health Literacy in Adults (TOFHLA) is a functional literacy assessment tool that

Figure 2-1. Standardized Literacy Testing Worksheet

Fill out this worksheet to get a clear idea of all the elements that will be involved in your testing project. You can apply your answers from the first section to help analyze the criteria in the grid that follows.

Project Considerations

What do we want this information for? _____

What patient population are we studying? _____

Does this population have any physical (for example, poor hearing, failing vision, known illness) or cognitive liabilities that we should plan for? _____

Is this population English proficient? _____

Where will we conduct the test? _____

How long will we have to administer the test? _____

Who will administer the test? _____

Who will input and analyze the data? _____

How will we maintain patient confidentiality? _____

Who will receive copies of the results? _____

Selection Grid

	Test 1 _____	Test 2 _____	Test 3 _____
Ease of use			
Ease of scoring			
Time required			
Available in Spanish			
Cost			
Tested for validity and reliability			
Suitability for patient population			
Suitability for project goal			

Source: Davis T., et al.: Literacy testing in health care research. In Schwartzberg J.G., VanGeest J.B., Wang C.C. (eds.): *Understanding Health Literacy: Implications for Medicine and Public Health.* Chicago: American Medical Association, 2005, p. 174.

tests patients' reading comprehension and numeracy skills (*see* Figure 2-3, pages 29–30). The reading section tests a patient's ability to read using real materials from health care settings. Passages are from instructions for preparation for an upper gastrointestinal series, the patient rights and responsibilities section of a Medicaid application, and a standard hospital informed consent form. The numeracy questions reproduce real-life situations in receiving, following, and paying for medication plans. Items in both sections are arranged in increasing levels of difficulty.[30]

The full-length version of the TOFHLA takes about 22 minutes to administer (100 possible points) and is usually used for research projects. The short version (S-TOFHLA) takes only about 7 minutes (36 possible points) and can be used to screen patients in clinical settings, health education programs, or research studies. Both versions are available in Spanish as well as English.[30] Although there is no separate adolescent version of the test, results from a pilot test in which the TOFHLA was administered to a group of 50 teens suggested that the reading component is valid for this group as well.[31]

In all versions, patients receive one point for each correct answer. Scores are divided into adequate, marginal, and inadequate functional health literacy categories. Patients with adequate skills should be able to read and interpret most health care–related materials; those with marginal skills will probably have difficulty with these materials; and people with inadequate skills will not be able to use such materials at all.[30]

Figure 2-2. Rapid Estimate of Adult Literacy in Medicine (REALM) Word List

Reading Level _____

Patient Name _____ Date of Birth _____ Grade Completed _____

Date _____ Clinic _____ Examiner _____

List 1		List 2		List 3	
fat	____	fatigue	____	allergic	____
flu	____	pelvic	____	menstrual	____
pill	____	jaundice	____	testicle	____
dose	____	infection	____	colitis	____
eye	____	exercise	____	emergency	____
stress	____	behavior	____	medication	____
smear	____	prescription	____	occupation	____
nerves	____	notify	____	sexually	____
germs	____	gallbladder	____	alcoholism	____
meals	____	calories	____	irritation	____
disease	____	depression	____	constipation	____
cancer	____	miscarriage	____	gonorrhea	____
caffeine	____	pregnancy	____	inflammatory	____
attack	____	arthritis	____	diabetes	____
kidney	____	nutrition	____	hepatitis	____
hormones	____	menopause	____	antibiotics	____
herpes	____	appendix	____	diagnosis	____
seizure	____	abnormal	____	potassium	____
bowel	____	syphilis	____	anemia	____
asthma	____	hemorrhoids	____	obesity	____
rectal	____	nausea	____	osteoporosis	____
incest	____	directed	____	impetigo	____

SCORE
List 1 _____
List 2 _____
List 3 _____
Raw Score _____

Source: Copyright © Davis, Crouch, and Long. Used with permission.

Patients read these words aloud from a laminated list (which is also available in a larger font) and are given a point for each word they get right. The "raw score" is used to determine the patient's reading grade level. 0–18 = third grade or below; 19–44 = fourth to sixth grade; 45–60 = seventh to eighth grade; and 61–66 = ninth grade or above.

Newest Vital Sign

The Newest Vital Sign (NVS) consists of a nutrition label from a container of ice cream. You give this to the patient and ask him or her six questions based on the information on the label (*see* Figure 2-4, page 32). The tool takes only about three minutes to administer, and the quantitative nature of the questions means that you test both reading comprehension and mathematical ability at the same time.[32] As with the other tests, patients receive one point for each correct answer. A score of 4 or more indicates adequate literacy, 2 or 3 indicates limited literacy, and less than 2 means the patient has a better than 50% chance of marginal or inadequate literacy.[33]

As with the TOFHLA, the NVS is available in both English and Spanish versions.

Figure 2-3. Excerpts from the Test of Functional Health Literacy in Adults (TOFHLA)

Numeracy
Prompt 1

GARFIELD IM   16 Apr 93
FF941858 Dr. LUBIN, MICHAEL
PENICILLIN VK
250MG 40/0
Take one tablet by mouth four
times a day
02   (4 of 40)

If you take your first tablet at 7:00 A.M., when should you take the next one? _____

And the next one after that? _____

What about the last one for the day, when should you take that one? _____

Prompt 10

You can get care at no cost if after deductions your monthly income and other resources are less than:

$581 for a family of one $1,196 for a family of four
$786 for a family of two $1,401 for a family of five
$991 for a family of three $1,196 for a family of six

Let's say that after deductions, your monthly income and other resources are $1,129. And let's say you have 3 children. Would you have to pay for your care at that clinic?

Reading Comprehension
PASSAGE A: X-RAY PREPARATION

You must have an _____ stomach when you come for _____.
         a. asthma   a. is
         b. empty   b. an
         c. incest   c. if
         d. anemia   d. it

<u>The Day of the X-ray</u>

Do not eat _____.
         a. appointment
         b. walk-in
         c. breakfast
         d. clinic

If you have any _____, call the X-ray _____ at 616-4500.
         a. answers   a. Department
         b. exercises   b. Sprain
         c. tracts   c. Pharmacy
         d. questions   d. Toothache

(continued on page 31)

Figure 2-3. Excerpts from the Test of Functional Health Literacy in Adults (TOFHLA) (continued)

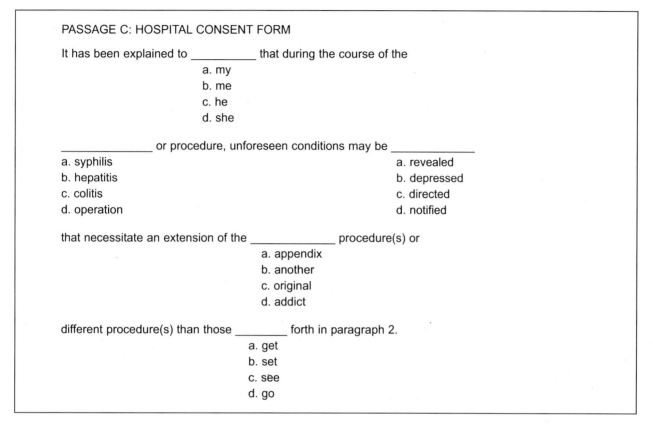

PASSAGE C: HOSPITAL CONSENT FORM

It has been explained to _____ that during the course of the
            a. my
            b. me
            c. he
            d. she

_____ or procedure, unforeseen conditions may be _____
a. syphilis   a. revealed
b. hepatitis   b. depressed
c. colitis   c. directed
d. operation   d. notified

that necessitate an extension of the _____ procedure(s) or
                        a. appendix
                        b. another
                        c. original
                        d. addict

different procedure(s) than those _____ forth in paragraph 2.
                        a. get
                        b. set
                        c. see
                        d. go

Source: Used with permission from Peppercorn Books and Press, Inc.

These questions show how the TOFHLA can be used to test adult patients for numeracy and reading comprehension skills. For each numeracy item, the patient is handed a "prompt," such as a mock prescription label or a text passage, and instructed to read it silently. The person administering the test then asks the questions shown. For reading comprehension, different types of instructions are given in the form of sentences with words missing. Under each blank line for a missing word, four possible choices are given to complete the sentence. The patient is asked to complete each passage.

Other Tests

Many other standard testing tools are available. For example, the Wide Range Achievement Test–Revised 3 (WRAT-R3) can be used to test reading, spelling, and mathematical abilities. The reading subtest is a word recognition test, similar to the REALM. Although the WRAT-R3 is designed for use with both children and adults and can be given in three to five minutes, the words in the reading section can be difficult for administrators and patients with reading levels below ninth grade.[17]

Tests for individual conditions and diseases have also been created, generally based on either the REALM or the TOFHLA. The Literacy Assessment for Diabetes, a word-recognition test modeled on the REALM, uses 60 terms frequently heard by people living with diabetes (such as *snack* and *retinopathy*).[17] The Nutritional Literacy Scale, modeled after the reading comprehension section of the S-TOFHLA, was developed for research in such areas as obesity, hypertension, and diabetes to test patients' literacy skills as they apply to nutritional concepts.[34]

Figure 2-4. The Newest Vital Sign Label and Questionnaire

Nutrition Facts	
Serving Size	½ cup
Servings per container	4

Amount per serving			
Calories 250		Fat Cal	120
			%DV
Total Fat 13g			20%
Sat Fat 9g			40%
Cholesterol 28mg			12%
Sodium 55mg			2%
Total Carbohydrate 30g			12%
Dietary Fiber 2g			
Sugars 23g			
Protein 4g			8%

*Percentage Daily Values (DV) are based on a 2,000 calorie diet. Your daily values may be higher or lower depending on your calorie needs.
Ingredients: Cream, Skim Milk, Liquid Sugar, Water, Egg Yolks, Brown Sugar, Milkfat, Peanut Oil, Sugar, Butter, Salt, Carrageenan, Vanilla Extract.

Score Sheet for the Newest Vital Sign Questions and Answers

READ TO SUBJECT: This information is on the back of a container of a pint of ice cream.

ANSWER CORRECT? yes no

1. If you eat the entire container, how many calories will you eat?
   Answer: 1,000 is the only correct answer

2. If you are allowed to eat 60 grams of carbohydrates as a snack, how much ice cream could you have?
   Answer: Any of the following is correct: 1 cup (or any amount up to 1 cup), Half the container Note: If patient answers "two servings," ask "How much ice cream would that be if you were to measure it into a bowl."

3. Your doctor advises you to reduce the amount of saturated fat in your diet. You usually have 42 g of saturated fat each day, which includes one serving of ice cream. If you stop eating ice cream, how many grams of saturated fat would you be consuming each day?
   Answer: 33 is the only correct answer

4. If you usually eat 2500 calories in a day, what percentage of your daily value of calories will you be eating if you eat one serving?
   Answer: 10% is the only correct answer

READ TO SUBJECT: Pretend that you are allergic to the following substances: Penicillin, peanuts, latex gloves, and bee stings.

5. Is it safe for you to eat this ice cream?
   Answer: No

6. (Ask only if the patient responds "no" to question 5): Why not?
   Answer: Because it has peanut oil.

Interpretation   Number of correct answers:

Score of 0-1 suggests high likelihood (50% or more) of limited literacy
Score of 2-3 indicates the possibility of limited literacy.
Score of 4-6 almost always indicates adequate literacy.

Source: © Pfizer. Reproduced with permission.

The patient refers to the nutritional label from an ice cream container (left) *to answer the six questions posed by the person administering the test* (right). *The patient should not be given time to review the label prior to the questions being asked.*

One team of researchers came up with a literacy test in Spanish that builds on the REALM's example. For the Short Assessment of Health Literacy for Spanish-Speaking Adults (SAHLSA), the terms from the REALM were translated into Spanish; patients are asked to read each word aloud and then think of another word that means roughly the same thing to demonstrate comprehension. The test takes only three to six minutes and can be used to assess individual or community literacy levels. However, the different idioms used by people from various Latin American countries may pose a problem for the comprehension section.[35]

Gathering Population-Level Information

If your organization has opted to forgo standardized testing, you can still estimate your patient population's average health literacy level by using one of the online calculators that analyze age, race, ethnicity, English proficiency, and Medicaid status percentages for your community and then approximate the percentage of people who may have low health literacy.[8,36] For example, Pfizer's Prevalence Calculator, which is available for free download (http://www.pfizerhealthliteracy.com/physicians-providers/prevalence-calculator.html), uses a simple formula and data from the health literacy component of the NAAL to determine how many people in your population are at risk. Because these estimates are for the general population, they cannot be applied to individual patients, but they can guide your organization's overall health literacy efforts.

Possible Links Between Written and Oral Literacy

All of the assessment tools discussed in this section deal with health literacy as it applies to written materials. According to Baker, it is likely that people with low print health literacy will also have low oral health literacy, because the mental processes for understanding both written and spoken words are closely related. However, there is currently no test to gauge a person's oral health literacy level.[37]

Collecting Data for Health Literacy

Although the Health Research and Educational Trust reports that 52% of hospitals collect information on patients' primary language to include in the medical record, only 20% gather data about patients' literacy levels.[23] The Joint Commission's HLC study found that about 75% or more of participating hospitals collect data on patient race, primary language, and religion, and they have various ways of identifying patients' linguistic and cultural needs.[11]

Health care organizations do automatically collect information on health literacy, but research studies increase our understanding of the association between literacy levels and specific diseases or conditions. One study conducted as part of the Vermont Diabetes Information System looked at how many adults with diabetes and heart failure had limited literacy. Research assistants conducted home interviews with a random sample of patients from 73 primary care practices in Vermont and northern New Hampshire and New York. These interviews included the collection of demographic data and the administration of a standardized literacy test. Results from the study showed that 27% of patients with diabetes and heart failure had limited literacy. The association was not significant after adjustments for education level were made, but the numbers indicated that clinicians need to be aware that many

patients have literacy limitations that can affect their use of written materials.[38]

Data can also be used to identify correlations between health literacy and patients' use of health services. For example, the health literacy of low-income Latinas aged 40 to 78 who attended two women's health services centers in New York was assessed, along with the patients' knowledge of and behaviors associated with cervical cancer screening. Interviewers used the Spanish version of the TOFHLA. Women with inadequate health literacy were significantly less likely than those with marginal or adequate health literacy to have ever had a Pap smear.[39]

Whether or not you use a standardized test to gather data on your patients' health literacy levels, there are other data categories that relate to various aspects of health literacy and patient-centered care. Researchers who assessed culturally competent care from the patient perspective recommended that health care facilities and systems continually monitor their patient populations through quantitative and qualitative data collection. These data should include patients' race or ethnicity, socioeconomic status, English proficiency, and preferred language or language spoken at home, health literacy, and use of complementary and alternative medical practices.[40]

You may use a variety of instruments to gather information. For example, you might modify your registration forms to capture demographic data,[40] and your assessment forms could include basic health literacy–related questions and use of alternative therapies. You could also get feedback on patient understanding of both verbal and written health information through surveys, focus groups, comment cards, or telephone hotlines.[41] Researchers in Australia used in-depth, loosely structured interviews to gather qualitative data from adults of various literacy levels about their views concerning patient decision aids used for colorectal cancer screening.[42]

Formal collection and analysis of data pertaining to both your patients' health literacy needs and your efforts to meet those needs are just as important as the collection and analysis of every other type of data in your organization. Knowing the cultural backgrounds, preferred languages, and literacy levels of your main population(s) allows you to assess your communication and educational processes for opportunities to improve. Getting support for health literacy activities is usually easier when you can show leaders and staff quantitative evidence of the need for change. For example, tracking wait times for interpreters in your organization may show that you need to hire more staff in this area; the percentage of certain preferred patient languages and the number of calls made to a telephone interpreter service for the same languages may indicate that you need to add in-house interpreters for those languages.

Ongoing monitoring of patient demographics and processes is also important. The ratio of different racial and ethnic groups fluctuates constantly, particularly in heavily populated areas, and this can affect the appropriateness of your language and translation services, health literacy programs, educational offerings, and so on. Even with careful planning, revisions to existing processes can sometimes have unexpected consequences, and you need to continue to assess the performance of these processes to catch any problems as early as possible. Using patient outcomes as a performance measure to show the value of a health literacy program—for example, fewer emer-

gency department admissions for asthma patients who have received a new educational intervention and handouts that illustrate how to use an inhaler properly—can help you convince leaders to continue to allocate resources for these types of projects.

Nor is data collection for health literacy and related topics such as patient safety necessary only in the acute care setting. Effective communication and education is also crucial in ambulatory and home care. Patients need clear instructions about how to monitor their health status, evaluate and report changes, follow medication regimens, store and use medical equipment and supplies, and so on to achieve good outcomes. Staff in long term care organizations need to understand and be sensitive to the cultural, linguistic, and literacy needs of a population that usually has both physical and cognitive impairments, as well as family members who visit and help care for them.

After you have assessed the health literacy levels of your patients, you can evaluate your care delivery processes and materials to see whether they are in sync with those levels. Chapter 3 has suggestions for how to make your environment of care, communication methods, forms, and patient information more patient friendly.

References

1. Kutner M., et al.: *The Health Literacy of America's Adults: Results from the 2003 National Assessment of Adult Literacy.* NCES 2006-483. Washington, DC: U.S. Department of Education, National Center for Education Statistics, 2006.
2. Freudenberg N.: Reframing school dropout as a public health issue. *Prev Chronic Dis* 4:1–11, Oct. 2007.
3. Davis T.C., et al.: The role of inadequate health literacy skills in colorectal cancer screening. *Cancer Invest* 19(2): 193–200, 2001.
4. Canadian Council on Learning: *Adult Literacy: A Synthesis of Evidence.* British Columbia Ministry of Advanced Education. May 6, 2006. http://www.aved.gov.bc.ca/ccl_question_scans/documents/Adult_Literacy .pdf (accessed Dec. 30, 2008).
5. Mayer G.G.: How eliminating communications roadblocks helps patients manage chronic illness. *HealthLeaders News,* Mar. 6, 2007. http://www.healthleadersmedia.com/print.cfm?content_id=87597&parent=105 (accessed Dec. 30, 2008).
6. Rao P.R.: Health literacy: The cornerstone of patient safety. *ASHA Leader* 12:8–9, 20, May 8, 2007.
7. Brown H., et al.: *Literacy of Older Adults in America: Results from the National Adult Literacy Survey.* Washington, DC: U.S. Department of Education, 1996.
8. American Medical Association: *Improving Communication—Improving Care: An Ethical Force Program™ Consensus Report.* Chicago: American Medical Association, 2006.
9. U.S. Department of Health & Human Services, Office of Minority Health: *Asian American/Pacific Islander Profile.* http://www.omhrc.gov/templates/browse.aspx?lvl=2&lvlID=53 (accessed Dec. 30, 2008).
10. U.S. Census Bureau: *Census 2000 Summary File 3.* http://www.census.gov/Press-Release/www/2002/sumfile3.html (accessed Dec. 30, 2008).
11. Wilson-Stronk A., Galvez E.: The Joint Commission: *Hospitals, Language, and Culture: A Snapshot of the Nation.* Oakbrook Terrace, IL: The Joint Commission, 2007.
12. U.S. Census Bureau: *2005-2007 American Community Survey 3-Year Estimates.* http://factfinder.census.gov (accessed Feb. 23, 2009).
13. Joint Commission Resources: *Providing Culturally and Linguistically Competent Health Care.* Oakbrook Terrace, IL: Joint Commission Resources, 2006.
14. Shaw S.J., et al.: The role of culture in health literacy and chronic disease screening and management. *J Immigr Minor Health,* Apr. 1, 2008. [Epub]
15. Sarkar U., et. al.: Use of an interactive, telephone-based self-management support program to identify adverse events among ambulatory diabetes patients. *J Gen Intern Med* 23(4):459–465, 2007.
16. Riley J.B., Cloonan P., Norton C.: Low health literacy: A challenge to critical care. *Crit Care Nurs Q* 29(2):174–178, 2006.
17. Davis T., et al.: Literacy testing in health care research. In Schwartzberg J.G., VanGeest J.B., Wang C.C. (eds.): *Understanding Health Literacy: Implications for Medicine and Public Health.* Chicago: American Medical Association, 2005, pp. 157–179.
18. Weiss B.D.: *Health Literacy and Patient Safety: Help Patients Understand. Manual for Clinicians,* 2nd ed. Chicago: American Medical Association Foundation and American Medical Association, 2007.
19. Davidson D.A.: Health literacy: Adverse implications for patients and physicians. *J Med Pract Manage* 19:207–210, Jan.–Feb. 2004.
20. Wallace L.S., et al.: Can screening items identify surgery patients at risk of limited health literacy? *J Surg Res* 140:208–213, 2007.
21. Bevan J.L., Pecchioni L.L.: Understanding the impact of family caregiver cancer literacy on patient health outcomes. *Patient Educ Couns* 71:356–364, 2008.
22. Persell S.D., et al.: Limited health literacy is a barrier to medication reconciliation in ambulatory care. *J Gen Intern Med* 22(11):1523–1526, 2007.
23. The Joint Commission: *"What Did the Doctor Say?" Improving Health Literacy to Protect Patient Safety* (white paper). Oakbrook Terrace, IL: 2007.
24. Lehna C., McNeil J.: Mixed-methods exploration of parents' health information understanding. *Clin Nurs Res* 17:133–144, May 2008.
25. Baker D.W.: Development of a brief test to measure functional health literacy. *Patient Educ Couns* 38:33–42, 1999.
26. Doak C.C., Doak L.G., Root J.H.: *Teaching Patients with Low Literacy Skills,* 2nd ed. Philadelphia: J. B. Lippincott Company, 1996.
27. Davis T., et al.: *Rapid Estimate of Adult Literacy in Medicine: Administration Manual.* Shreveport, LA: Prevention and Patient Education Project, LSU Health Sciences Center, n.d.
28. Arozullah A.M., et al.: Development and validation of a short-form, rapid estimate of adult literacy in medicine. *Med Care* 45:1026–1033, Nov. 2007.
29. Davis T., et al.: *Rapid Estimate of Adolescent Literacy in Medicine (REALM-Teen): Administration Manual.* Shreveport, LA: LSU Health Sciences Center, Department of Pediatrics, n.d.
30. Nurss J.R., et al.: *TOFHLA: Test of the Functional Health Literacy in Adults.* Snow Camp, NC: Peppercorn Books & Press Inc., Jan. 2001.
31. Chisolm D.J., Buchanan L.: Measuring adolescent functional health literacy: A pilot validation of the Test of Functional Health Literacy in Adults. *J Adolesc Health* 41:312–314, 2007.
32. Monachos C.L.: Assessing and addressing low health literacy among surgical outpatients. *AORN J* 86:373–383, Sep. 2007.
33. Weiss B.D., et al.: Quick assessment of literacy in primary care: The Newest Vital Sign. *Ann Fam Med* 3:514–522, Nov.–Dec. 2005.
34. Diamond J.J.: Development of a reliable and construct valid measure of nutritional literacy in adults. *Nutr J* 6, Feb. 14, 2007. http://www.nutritionj.com/content/6/1/5 (accessed Dec. 30, 2008).
35. Lee S-Y.D., et al.: Development of an easy-to-use Spanish health literacy test. *Health Serv Res* 41(pt. I):1392–1412, Aug. 2006.
36. Larson L.: Health literacy: How are your patients reading you? *Trustee* pp. 8–12, May 2007.
37. Baker D.W.: The meaning and the measure of health literacy. *J Gen Intern Med* 21:878–883, 2006.
38. Laramee A.S., Morris N., Littenberg B.: Relationship of literacy and heart failure in adults with diabetes. *BMC Fam Pract* 7:98–103, Jul. 2, 2007.
39. Garbers S., Chiasson M.A.: Inadequate functional health literacy in Spanish as a barrier to cervical cancer screening among immigrant Latinas in New York City. *Prev Chronic Dis,* Oct. 2004. http://www.cdc.gov/Pcd/issues/2004/oct/03_0038.htm (accessed Dec. 30, 2008).
40. Ngo-Metzger Q., et al.: Providing high-quality care for limited English proficient patients: The importance of language concordance and interpreter use. *J Gen Intern Med* 22(suppl. 2):324–330, 2007.
41. Kreps G.L., Sparks L.: Meeting the health literacy needs of immigrant populations. *Patient Educ Couns* 71:328–332, 2008.
42. Smith S.K., et al.: Information needs and preferences of low and high literacy consumers for decisions about colorectal cancer screening: Utilizing a linguistic model. *Health Expect* 11:123–136, 2008.

CHAPTER 3

IMPLEMENTING SOLUTIONS

Identifying vulnerable populations and those at risk for low health literacy levels does no good if the information is not used to make improvements throughout the health care facility or system. This chapter outlines strategies for making an organizationwide push for better health literacy, improving everyone's communication skills, and providing reliable health information to anyone who needs it.

Getting Everyone Involved

Good communication is a team effort, and every member of the organization from the admission/intake staff and receptionist to the nurses, physicians, pharmacists, and therapists to educators, social workers, and transport personnel to leaders and board members needs to know about and help alleviate the health literacy challenges facing your patients.

Making Health Literacy a Priority

As with any improvement project, a health literacy program needs commitment from leadership to succeed. Although many activities may begin as grassroots efforts, they can go only so far without support from the top. Besides the need for resources to move projects forward, consideration of health literacy needs to be incorporated into organizational policies and procedures so it does not get lost among other priorities. In a struggling economy with ever-increasing regulatory requirements, it is easy for education and other health literacy–related areas to end up at the bottom of an organization's to-do list, but the consequences of not addressing the gaps in patients' understanding and knowledge can lead to greater costs in medical errors, poor patient outcomes, more clinic visits or hospital readmissions, longer lengths of stay,

emergency calls for home health nurses (contributing to staffing problems), and so on.

Your leaders can demonstrate their commitment to health literacy by mandating training in better patient communication techniques for everyone in the organization—leaders, health care professionals, and support staff alike. If you sponsor or conduct seminars, conventions, health fairs, or similar events, leaders can dedicate sessions or space to raising both providers' and patients' awareness of health literacy issues. Leaders can also build relationships with community health leaders, policymakers, and educators to encourage collaboration on providing the local population with useful, understandable health information.

Health literacy affects all areas of your organization, so try to incorporate it into all strategic plans. For example, you might establish a policy that all materials that go to the public—educational brochures, forms, press releases, surveys, and so on—from any part of your organization will be written to a certain grade level and translated into the languages most prevalent among your patient population. As policymakers and insurers become more aware of the mismatch between current medical information and patients' understanding, they will also become more interested in holding providers responsible for better communication. Including health literacy in grant proposals and funding requests will demonstrate your commitment to addressing this issue. You can also build a health literacy database for your organization's intranet or have materials about health literacy and communication available in your facility's resource center so staff have easy access to references and information.

If you are having trouble finding ways to integrate health literacy efforts into normal operations, the sample action plan for improving health literacy from the Office of Disease Prevention and Health Promotion may give you some ideas (http://www.health.gov/ communication/ literacy/sampleplan.htm) (*see* Figure 3-1, pages 39–40). The plan includes a problem statement followed by priorities, each of which has its own objective and set of proposed actions. The five priorities include incorporating health literacy improvement into the organization's mission, planning, and evaluation; planning for the design and assessment of materials, messages, and resources that go to patients; and supporting health literacy research, training, and practice.[1] The last item highlights the importance of making sure all staff are educated to help patients with poor health literacy wherever they may be in the care continuum.

Educating Staff

Just as you need to have ongoing data collection for your health literacy activities, staff need ongoing education. Shifts in populations, community growth, and staff turnover mean that training needs to be done at regular intervals to keep everyone's skills current. Instruction about health literacy issues, ways to identify patients who may need extra help, and effective communication techniques should be included in new employee orientation, reviewed in staff meetings, and updated in seminars and in-services.

No one should be left out of training, because everyone in your organization may come into contact with patients and families. For instance, a lab technician or your CEO may find a visitor wandering the halls near the cafeteria and trying to find his or her way back to a patient room. Office staff in a home care agency may need to talk to patients or family members over the phone about scheduling, billing, insurance, and so on. Workers on the front lines need to know how to access language services for patients with limited English proficiency (LEP).

Involving patients in training by having them talk to different groups about difficulties they have experienced in the care process can bring the need for better communication home. It can also motivate everyone involved to put extra effort into behaviors such as watching for nonverbal cues that may signal a need for help or offering to help patients before they need to ask. Health professionals who provide specific medical information, such as physicians, nurses, and pharmacists, need to learn how to adapt their delivery for patients who may have trouble understanding. In addition, a wealth of materials is available online to use in training. (*See* the Appendix for a sample of tools and training resources.) To ensure that everyone in the organization understands the importance of communicating clearly, you may choose to include health literacy knowledge and effective communication methods in job descriptions, competency requirements, and annual performance evaluations.

Creating an Environment That Promotes Good Communication

Just as entering a health care setting or making an appointment with a physician can be an intimidating prospect for people with low health literacy. They know they will have to find their way around the facility, explain their symptoms, and fill out forms—all before the actual examination takes place and they are called on to try to interpret whatever the physician tells them. Then there can be the confusion of a new medication or proposed lifestyle changes, diagnostic procedures, treatments ranging from physical therapy to surgery, and so on. The fear associated with being injured or ill is exacerbated by the anxiety of not being able to understand signs or verbal instructions and being afraid or ashamed to ask for help. Organizations can create an environment that will help patients feel more comfortable and will make care encounters less daunting so patients will be more willing and able to participate in their own care.

Understanding the Patient's Perspective

Chapter 2 discussed the importance of knowing your patient population and identifying groups that are at higher risk for poor health literacy. However, understanding the basic characteristics of your patients does not mean that you have grasped the full implications of those characteristics. Rima Rudd, M.S.P.H., Sc.D., defines the patient perspective as a combination of the patient's experience of the literacy-related demands con-

Figure 3-1. Sample Action Plan for Incorporating Health Literacy into Your Mission and Goals

Sample Action Plan to Improve Health Literacy

Following is a sample Action Plan to Improve Health Literacy for a fictional organization—ABC Community Health Center. The plan can be used as a guide for national, state, county, and community health organizations committed to improving health literacy. The sample plan includes both Action Steps and specific measurable objectives to be used for evaluation. Consider writing, adopting, and implementing a similar plan in your own organization.

ABC Community Health Center Action Plan

The Action Plan to Improve Health Literacy is a set of health literacy priorities to be addressed by the ABC Community Health Center. Health literacy is the degree to which individuals have the capacity to obtain, process, and understand basic health information and services needed to make appropriate health decisions. As one of ABC County's principle organizations for protecting the health of its citizens, the ABC Community Health Center is a critical agent for improving health literacy.

Statement of the Problem:
- Nine out of 10 adults may lack the skills needed to manage their health and prevent disease, according to the National Assessment of Adult Literacy.
- Limited health literacy has negative implications for health outcomes, health care quality, and health care costs.
- ABC County residents have diverse information needs, including those related to cultural differences, language, age, ability, and literacy skills, that affect their ability to obtain, process, and understand health information and services.
- There are numerous barriers to effective communication between ABC Community Health Center professionals and the public.

ABC Community Health Center Response:
The ABC Community Health Center, in accordance with its mission, will develop, implement, and evaluate programs and provide resources to improve health literacy. Health Center responsibilities include ensuring that health professionals can obtain and provide the public with accurate and appropriate health information. The ABC Community Health Center will strive to address the following five health literacy priorities:

Priority 1: Incorporate health literacy improvement in mission, planning, and evaluation.
Action Steps:
- <u>Identify specific programs and projects affected by limited health literacy</u>. Examine the ways in which health literacy activities can improve the effectiveness of these programs.
- <u>Include specific goals and objectives related to improving health literacy</u> in the Health Center's strategic plans, performance plans, and educational initiatives.
- <u>Include health literacy improvement in program evaluation criteria and itemize health literacy improvement in budget requests</u>.

Objective: Complete organizational health literacy "adult" for review by December. Identify the ways in which addressing health literacy can improve program effectiveness.

Priority 2: Support health literacy research, evaluation, training, and practice.
Action Steps:
- <u>Identify health literacy improvement in grants and contracts</u>. Recommend that all products be written in plain language and tested with the intended users. Encourage contractors and grantees to indicate and evaluate how their activities contribute to improved health literacy.
- <u>Incorporate health literacy research and evaluation results</u> in the development of practices/programs.
- <u>Include health literacy improvement in training and orientation</u>. Incorporate health literacy improvement into existing training materials for staff, grantees, and contractors. Post and share health literacy resources.

(continued on page 40)

Figure 3-1. Sample Action Plan for Incorporating Health Literacy into Your Mission and Goals (continued)

Objective: Include an explicit reference to health literacy, where appropriate, in at least 25% of community grants issued in current fiscal year.

Priority 3: Conduct formative, process, and outcome evaluation to design and assess materials, messages, and resources.

Action Steps:

- Identify the intended users. Segment users based on epidemiologic characteristics, demographics, literacy skills, behavior, culture, beliefs, knowledge, attitudes, and other factors.
- Acknowledge and respect cultural differences. Cultural factors include, but are not limited to, race, ethnicity, language, nationality, beliefs, values, customs, religion, age, ability, gender, sexual orientation, socioeconomic status, occupation, housing status, and regional differences.
- Use plain language. Break complex information into understandable chunks, define technical terms, and use an active voice.
- Apply user-centered design principles, including iterative testing, to the creation of new materials, including content on the Web.

Objective: For all new public education initiatives launched after January:

Conduct formative evaluation 100% of the time.
Conduct process evaluation 90% of the time.
Conduct outcome evaluation 60% of the time.

Priority 4: Enhance dissemination of timely, accurate, and appropriate health information to health professionals and the public.

Action Steps:

- Identify and/or develop appropriate methods for information dissemination. Consider a wide variety of dissemination methods that could improve people's ability to obtain reliable and relevant health information, particularly for members of minority populations.
- Collaborate with adult educators, journalists, and other nontraditional partners to increase the dissemination of health information to the community.

Objective: Cosponsor, implement, and evaluate two public education activities with nontraditional partners in the community in current fiscal year.

Priority 5: Design health literacy improvements to health care and public health systems that enhance access to health services.

Action Steps:

- Improve the usability of medical forms and instructions. Write or rewrite forms to ensure clarity and simplicity. Test forms with intended users and revise as needed. Provide forms, signs, and services in multiple languages.
- Support health literacy and cultural competency training for health professionals in the community, including health care providers and public health officials.

Objective: Install new easy-to-understand signage in more than one language inside and outside the Community Health Center by December.

Source: Office of Disease Prevention and Health Promotion, U.S. Department of Health & Human Services.

Developed for a theoretical community health center, the priorities and actions in this plan are general and can be adapted for any setting.

Starting Early

Both the American Medical Association and the Institute of Medicine support incorporating health literacy training into all medical and health professional schools' curricula.[2,3] Highlighting the importance of good patient-physician communication, the United States Medical Licensing Examination requires that between the third and fourth years of medical school, students complete a clinical skills examination to evaluate their ability to gather information, perform physical exams, and communicate findings to standardized patients.[4]

Two medical schools in Chicago have responded to the demand for early training by embedding and integrating health literacy issues into required courses. The University of Chicago Pritzker School of Medicine's health literacy curriculum spans the first three years of medical school; that of Northwestern University's Feinberg School of Medicine spans the first year. Both programs are designed to improve student awareness of how low literacy affects health, health care, and medical encounters. The focus on clear communication and strategies to ensure patient understanding is intended to enhance students' ability to interact effectively with all patients. The reasoning behind this approach is that if training focuses first on identifying individuals with limited literacy and then using additional communication tools specifically for them, providers may begin to avoid these patients because of the potential increase in work load and cost. Whereas teaching effective communication techniques, such as using plain language and teach-back, for use with all patients makes health care disparities less likely.[5]

fronted in health care settings and the sense of adequacy or inadequacy he or she feels because of those demands.[6] It is important to take the information you already have about your population and build a profile of your patients' needs. For example, if you serve a diverse community, you might ask yourself the following questions about each cultural group[7]:

➤ What language is most commonly spoken by this group?

➤ What cultural or religious beliefs may affect care (for example, fasting or requiring female practitioners for female patients)?

➤ What are the common dietary practices that can affect care (such as vegetarianism)?

➤ How do members of this group prefer to communicate (for instance, avoiding eye contact)?

➤ How do they view illness, medical treatment, and death?

Some organizations use "cultural brokers" such as chaplains, language services departments, or nurses who have been trained in transcultural care to help providers understand how patients' religious and cultural beliefs can influence their understanding and acceptance of proposed treatments.[7]

When you have a good idea of the needs of your different populations, try putting yourself in their shoes. A good way to examine your environment is by pretending you are a patient and following the same processes and routes as he or she would. Call your office or organization for an appointment or a test. Does a person answer, or do you have to press a number of selections in an automated menu before you get to someone? How simple is the appointment procedure? Is there a system to call patients the day before their appointment to remind them of the time and any preparations they need to make?

Next, enter your organization and try to see it as though for the first time. Are signs understandable to people without medical knowledge (for example, many will not guess that *oncology* refers to cancer) or with poor English skills or failing eyesight? Are receptionists or front office staff proactive about greeting and offering to help you? How complicated is the sign-in or admission process? How many forms do you need to fill out? Are they redundant? Does someone offer to help you with the forms? Is an interpreter available if you need one? Would you feel comfortable asking questions?

The best source of information about your care environment is patients. Look at the feedback given on survey forms for clues about where processes get bogged down. Solicit opinions informally at different points in

Figure 3-2. How Patient Friendly Is Our Organization?

Telephone Contact

Calls are answered by a person rather than a machine. _____

When automated menus are used, they are simple to follow and are available in languages common to the patient population. _____

Office staff speak slowly and distinctly enough for callers to understand. _____

If staff do not speak the caller's language, interpretive services are available. _____

Staff ask for the least amount of information necessary. _____

Staff volunteer directions to the office/organization. _____

Staff explain any preparatory measures to be taken for the appointment (for example, bringing current medications to a physician visit, fasting before a blood test). _____

If time permits, directions and/or preparatory instructions are sent to the patient (e-mail, fax, or mail). _____

Reminder calls are placed to patients the day/night before their appointment. _____

Care Environment

Someone is available to greet patients as they enter and direct/take them to the appropriate department. _____

Receptionists/admissions staff are friendly and offer to help rather than wait for patients to ask. _____

Signs are large, use pictures, and are written in plain language. _____

The sign-in/admission process is as streamlined as possible to avoid redundant steps and forms. _____

Forms are simple to follow and use. _____

Forms are available in common languages and in large type for the vision impaired. _____

Staff offer to help patients fill out forms. _____

Interpreters are available for limited English proficiency (LEP) patients. _____

Staff encourage patients to ask questions about their care or any part of the process. _____

Sources: Rudd R.E., et al.: Literacy demands in health care settings: The patient perspective. In Schwartzberg J.G., VanGeest J.B., Wang C.C. (eds.): *Understanding Health Literacy: Implications for Medicine and Public Health*, Chicago: American Medical Association, 2005, pp. 69–84; Weiss B.D.: *Health Literacy and Patient Safety: Help Patients Understand. Manual for Clinicians*, 2nd ed. Chicago: American Medical Association Foundation and American Medical Association, 2007; Joint Commission Resources: *Providing Culturally and Linguistically Competent Health Care*. Oakbrook Terrace, IL: Joint Commission on Accreditation of Healthcare Organizations, 2006.

---

the care process, such as in the waiting room, at the conclusion of the discharge process, or in the pharmacy while prescriptions are being filled.

Use the checklist shown in Figure 3-2 (above) as a starting point for evaluating your facility on your own or with the help of your patients:

Empowering Patients

Patient-centered care focuses on involving patients in all aspects of the decision-making process as much as possible (and as far as they prefer to be involved). Feelings of being lost or helpless within a large, impersonal health care system are an obstacle to such involvement. Patients from minority or low-income groups are more likely to believe that their opinions and preferences in patient care are ignored. Similarly, many people who use complementary medicines, supplements, and alternative therapies are reluctant to admit this for fear that their choices will not be respected by those who practice traditional medicine.[8] Cognitive or physical impairments, poor language skills, and cultural barriers can make patients feel that they have no voice.

People with low literacy ask fewer questions. According to Terry Davis, Ph.D., Louisiana State University Health Sciences Center-Shreveport, "If someone's asked [for clarification] once and he or she is still not clear, it takes a very assertive person to say, 'I still don't understand what you're talking about.' This is true whether you're talking to your doctor, your lawyer, or your mechanic."

Table 3-1. Principles of the Speak Up™ Campaign

Speak up if you have questions or concerns, and if you don't understand, ask again. It's your body and you have a right to know.

Pay attention to the care you are receiving. Make sure you're getting the right treatments and medications by the right health care professionals. Don't assume anything.

Educate yourself about your diagnosis, the medical tests you are undergoing, and your treatment plan.

Ask a trusted family member or friend to be your advocate.

Know what medications you take and why you take them. Medication errors are the most common health care mistakes.

Use a hospital, clinic, surgery center, or other type of health care organization that has undergone a rigorous on-site evaluation against established, state-of-the-art quality and safety standards, such as that provided by The Joint Commission.

Participate in all decisions about your treatment. You are the center of the health care team.

Speak Up Initiatives

Speak Up Initiatives include the following:
- Help Prevent Errors in Your Care
- Help Avoid Mistakes in Your Surgery
- Information for Living Organ Donors
- Five Things You Can Do to Prevent Infection
- Help Avoid Mistakes with Your Medicines
- What You Should Know About Research Studies
- Planning Your Follow-up Care
- Help Prevent Medical Test Mistakes
- Know Your Rights
- Understanding Your Doctors and Other Caregivers
- What You Should Know About Pain Management

© The Joint Commission.

Several tools and initiatives are available to encourage patients to participate more fully in their care. The Joint Commission, with the Centers for Medicare & Medicaid Services (CMS), launched the national Speak Up™ campaign in 2002 to promote patients' role in preventing medical errors by being active, informed participants of the health care team (*see* Table 3-1, above). Brochures, posters, and buttons on patient safety topics such as preventing infections, knowing your rights, planning for follow-up care, and understanding caregivers raise both patient and provider awareness; the

information can be used in patient education materials, on Web sites, in community newsletters, at health fairs, and in staff training and orientation. Information about the campaign and Speak Up materials are available online as free downloads at http://www.jointcommission.org/ PatientSafety/SpeakUp. There are no copyright or reprinting permissions required for the Speak Up materials or copy. In references to the materials or copy, The Joint Commission asks to be credited as the source for the materials or copy.

In May 2003 the Partnership for Clear Health Communication launched its Ask Me 3™ campaign. The foundation of the Ask Me 3 tool is three questions that patients should ask during any health care encounter:

1. What is my main problem?
2. What do I need to do?
3. Why is it important for me to do this?

These questions provide an excellent guide for physicians and other health care professionals in structuring the information they provide. Many patients are not interested in how they acquired a condition or disease or what the specific anatomical consequences are. They want specific information about what to do to cure it or alleviate the symptoms and to know how their daily lives will be affected. You can find information about implementing Ask Me 3, as well as downloads of brochures and posters in English and Spanish, at http://www.npsf.org/askme3.

Patients also feel empowered when they know that their views are valued. Asking for and using their feedback when creating or revising forms and materials (discussed later in this chapter) or in evaluating your care environment, as mentioned earlier, lets patients know that they are an important part of the team and that their opinions are respected.

The most significant factor in patients' sense of empowerment may be the attitude of your staff and health care professionals. Displaying a willingness to listen, help, and encourage goes a long way toward establishing an environment of trust and mutual esteem.

Caution your staff against stereotyping patients based on race, gender, ethnicity, perceived income or educational level, and so on. Knowledge of cultural and language issues can give you helpful background information to consider during health care encounters, but each patient must be recognized as an individual with his or her own comfort level about the care experience.

Making Interpretative Services Available

An important part of empowering patients and improving care outcomes is providing language access (interpretive) services within your organization. Such services—which may be provided by qualified in-house staff, through a contract agency, or via a telephone- or Web-based service—are essential for communicating with LEP patients or with those who do not speak English at all. Qualified sign language interpreters are also needed to help the hearing impaired receive and understand information.

Many organizations and private practices do not see the need for interpretive services, but various regulatory requirements ensure that these services are available. The federal Civil Rights Act mandates that hospitals provide interpretive services to LEP patients and those with disabilities that inhibit their communication abilities.[4] The CMS requires that that all Medicare and Medicaid beneficiaries have access to interpreters, and the Joint Commission's standards state that communication with patients must be carried out in a manner they can understand, which includes its being presented in the language with which they are most comfortable.

Studies have shown the need for interpreters in order to help prevent medical errors and to improve patients' care experience. For example, research into adverse events reported in six hospitals across the country found that about 49% of such events involving LEP patients resulted in some sort of physical harm, but that physical harm was reported in only 29.5% of events involving English-speaking patients.[9] Another study of LEP Asian-American patients found that those who did not speak the same language as their physicians and who were not given the option of having an interpreter reported receiving less health education.[10]

Several barriers to the use of language access services are common in health care settings. The cost of maintaining such services can be high, particularly for private practices, and few states offer reimbursement for this cost. There is also a lack of standardization for the provision of interpreters within organizations, systems, and communities, so it is difficult to coordinate efforts and ensure that the same information is delivered in the same way across settings. Perhaps most pervasive is the ambivalence of practitioners. Interpretation in many organizations has traditionally been provided by family members or friends, bilingual volunteers from the community, or ad hoc staff members, and clinicians may see no reason to add a possibly time-consuming and certainly costly step to a process that they feel works fine as it is. Unfortunately, the use of untrained interpreters has many downfalls,[4,11] including the following:

➤ Information may be omitted or altered either intentionally or by accident.

➤ Interpreters who are not proficient in medical terminology can give incorrect information.

➤ Using unofficial interpreters can violate the privacy requirements stipulated in the Health Insurance Portability and Accountability Act of 1996 (HIPAA).

➤ Children may not be emotionally mature enough to understand or handle certain topics.

➤ Staff members may not always be able to leave their other duties.

Professionally trained medical interpreters can help avoid medical errors, increase understanding, and encourage patients to ask questions and volunteer information they might avoid in the presence of family members. Schools across the country now offer certification classes in medical interpretation and translation, and you will want to make sure that any in-house interpreters you hire or those contracted through an agency or service have proper qualifications. They should also receive orientation in all aspects of your organization's operations, including areas such as emergency preparedness, and be regularly evaluated for competency.

The way you structure your language access services will depend on the size of your organization, how many languages your populations commonly speak, the volume of patients and scope of services, and so on. For example, if your ambulatory clinic's primary LEP population is Hispanic, but your community has a growing number of Chinese residents, you may choose to have an in-house interpreter for Spanish and contract with an outside agency for Chinese language services. Or your rural hospital may have very few non-English-speaking patients each year and choose to subscribe to a Web-based interpreter service to cover such encounters. The options and combinations are many, so you can establish a program that meets both your patients' needs and your budget. When you have your program in place, you must also educate clinicians and staff on how and when to request interpreters, emphasizing the fact that any extra time taken will improve a patient's chances for positive outcomes.

Improving Signage

Finding a specific department in a health care organization can be difficult for anyone. The wording on signs may not match what people have been told to look for. For example, a man has been told by his physician that he needs "an MRI," but when he arrives at the hospital, he encounters a multitude of signs but none that say *MRI*. When he finally finds the outpatient registration desk, he is told that he needs the "nuclear medicine department." Interpreting staff members' instructions for navigating the corridors can also be challenging. Some organizations paint colored lines on the floor and tell patients to "Follow the blue line until it crosses the yellow line. Then follow the yellow line until you reach the red elevators." This method presumes that patients have good eyesight (with no color vision deficiencies), good memories, and good instincts for which line to follow when two lines of the same color intersect. Maps posted on walls at strategic points often display the same language as that used on signs, with symbols appearing only for points such as restrooms and emergency exits.

Many organizations tap volunteers from the community as guides for patients and visitors. Instead of relying on maps or verbal instructions, anyone entering the organization is greeted at a central point by a receptionist. After their destination is determined, whether it is registration, a diagnostic department, or a patient

room, they are taken there by a volunteer who is familiar with all areas of the building. All departments may call a central number for a guide and should be encouraged to do so. Staff often believe that patients who have been led to a certain area for testing or to a specific patient's room will be able to find their way back to the main entrance without help, but the return journey can be just as confusing as the initial one.

One way that has been proposed for making signage more accessible for staff and patients, particularly those who do not speak English, is the use of universal symbols, such as those used in airports and other public buildings. "Hablamos Juntos," a project aimed at improving patient-provider communications for Hispanics and funded by the Robert Wood Johnson Foundation, began exploring the use of symbols in health care signs in 2003. Its design team developed a set of 28 symbols that can be used in any health care setting (*see* Figure 3-3, page 46). Three hundred reviewers from four language groups—(1) English, (2) Spanish, (3) Indo-European, and (4) Asian—provided input on the symbols, and 17 of the 28 symbols were understood by at least 87% of the reviewers.[12] You can download the entire set of symbols and an implementation workbook from the "Hablamos Juntos" Web site (http://www.hablamos juntos.org/signage/symbols/default.symbols.asp#wus).

Symbols can preclude the need for translating signs into a variety of languages, or they can be added to clarify the language used. They can also be added to wall maps, handouts given to patients, and informational kiosks that use multimedia so posted signs match other written and graphic instructions. However, no matter how you choose to simplify the signage in your facility, the most commonly used resource for navigating your organization will still be staff members. Although the suggestions for better interpersonal communication in the next section are aimed primarily at clinicians and other health care professionals, they can be helpful for everyone in your organization.

Improving Face-to-Face Communication

Much of the important communication between

Figure 3-3. Universal Symbols for Health Care Signage

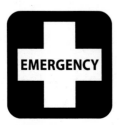

Emergency
Emergencia

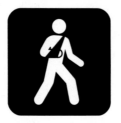

Outpatient
Paciente Ambulatorio

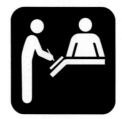

Registration
Registro

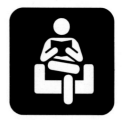

Waiting Area
Área de Espera

Source: © The Robert Wood Johnson Foundation. Used with permission.

You can use symbols such as these to help patients and visitors find key areas of your organization. The set of 28 symbols developed by Hablamos Juntos can be used in a variety of health care settings.

patients and members of the health care team takes place one-on-one: taking histories, discussing symptoms, explaining diagnoses, providing education and self-care instructions, consoling patients or family members. Effective communication is communication that is understood by both parties.[12] However, low health literacy, physical and cognitive problems, language barriers, and other factors can pose the following challenges to patients' comprehension[13]:

➤ They may not catch all information.

➤ They may have difficulty understanding the information presented.

➤ They may have trouble communicating the information to family members.

➤ They may find it difficult to recall what the practitioner said.

➤ They may find it difficult to recall what they said.

When health care professionals communicate well, patients experience less anxiety and better understanding, which in turn can lead to better compliance and outcomes.[14] In addition to training in cultural competency and the general needs of your populations, several techniques can help clinicians and staff build a rapport and talk more effectively with patients.

Using Plain Language

Any conversation requires a common language between participants. Unfortunately, many practitioners tend to use terms or words that people with low literacy find difficult to understand. To explain this concept to health professionals, Terry Davis uses the analogy of talking to your auto mechanic: "I don't know the right words to use to describe a problem to my mechanic. If you open the hood of my car, I can tell you where the battery is, but that's about it. A lot of people are that way when it comes to their bodies. I did some research about colon cancer several years ago, and many people didn't know what the term *screening* meant or understand the concept of looking for hidden cancer. They didn't know what or where their colon was, and nobody used the term *flexible sigmoidoscopy*."

When explaining conditions or treatments to patients, you need to avoid medical jargon and use the simplest terms possible. Table 3-2 (page 47) gives some examples of words that patients might find confusing and alternatives you may consider using.

You may also find it helpful to use the Ask Me 3 questions to structure your presentation of information and eliminate extraneous facts. For example, instead of giving a patient with a diagnosis of Type 2 diabetes the details of his or her test results and a long explanation of what hyperglycemia entails, you might begin the conversation in this manner:

You have diabetes. [What is my main problem?] *We're going to talk about what you eat and some medicines you*

Table 3-2. Terms Patients May Not Understand

Difficult Words	Possible Alternatives
Ailment	Illness, health problem, sickness
Benign	Is not cancer, will not cause harm
Chemotherapy	Drugs to treat cancer
Dysfunction	Problem
Hypertension	High blood pressure
Lesion	Infected patch of skin, sore, wound
Malignancy	Cancer
Oral	By mouth
Radiology	X-ray department
Toxic	Poisonous
Vertigo	Dizziness

Sources: Weiss B.D.: *Health Literacy and Patient Safety: Help Patients Understand. Manual for Clinicians,* 2nd ed. Chicago: American Medical Association Foundation and American Medical Association, 2007; Joint Commission Resources: Bear in mind the level of understanding during care—Standard RI.2.100. *The Joint Commission: The Source* 6:6, 7, 11, Feb. 2008.

can take to handle this. [What do I need to do?] *It is important to eat the right foods and take your medicine regularly to help you take care of your diabetes.* [Why is it important for me to do this?]

This basic information can then lead to further discussion about using a glucose meter to keep track of sugar levels and the possible side effects of hyper- and hypoglycemia.

Using Visual and Multimedia Aids

No matter how clearly you talk about a diagnosis or treatment plan, patients may need visual aids or multimedia tools to help them understand or drive the information home. You may decide to use models such as plaster casts of bones or pictures to illustrate your points. Even a simple sketch on the exam table paper may be helpful when illustrating a point or information about a particular condition. When choosing anatomical drawings or diagrams, make sure they are simple, are clearly labeled, and address only the areas that the patient needs to know for his or her specific condition. For example, if you are explaining what will happen during a colonoscopy, the accompanying drawing needs

to show only the colon and rectum; other organs such as the bladder or intestines are superfluous.

Using tools or devices that the patient will use as part of treatment can also be helpful. For instance, if you are explaining a drug regimen that includes several medications and requires strict adherence to a set schedule, you might want to have a weekly pill organizer on hand to show the patient how to divide up his or her medications and to use the organizer to make sure that all medicines have been taken. Most organizers have boxes with labels such as *Morning, Noon, Evening,* and *Bedtime* for each day, but patients can affix their own labels over these to indicate specific times.

You may want to have other media or recommendations for additional resources on hand to reinforce your message or to give patients additional information that they can explore at their leisure. CD-ROMs and audiotapes are good options because most people have some sort of audio system at home or in their cars. Videos and DVDs can explain diseases, testing, and treatment options; they are especially helpful in teaching or reminding patients how to perform tasks for self-care such as giving insulin injections or doing breast examinations. DVDs and CDs may also be used on a home computer or on a laptop in the health care setting to provide interactive education options.[14]

If your organization has a resource center or library, or if you know a patient has access to the Internet, you can recommend online resources for further research and learning. For example, MedlinePlus® (http://www.nlm.nih.gov/medlineplus) offers plain-language information as well as interactive tutorials on diseases, medicines, tests, and other health topics. Many Web sites offer information and instruction in several languages, which can be useful for LEP patients. Healthy Roads Media (http://www.healthyroadsmedia.org) allows you to download audio, multimedia, and written health education materials in 19 different languages, and LaRue Medical Literacy Learning Activities (http://mcedservices.com/medex/medex.htm), which help patients learn how to interpret labels and side effects of medications, are available in 5 languages.

Many government and professional organizations are working on their Web sites to make them more accessible to LEP patients, those with poor literacy, and those with limited computer skills. However, all Internet information is not created equal, and you should screen sites before you recommend them to patients. Questions to keep in mind as you review a site for reliability of information include the following[15]:

➤ Does the site verify and screen material?

➤ Are authors' credentials given?

➤ Is the publisher of the material listed?

➤ Is documentation consistently provided for statistics and statements?

➤ Is the information consistent with information from other sources?

You should also ask questions about how user-friendly the site is (see the discussion of developing Web sites later in this chapter for details). A medical or consumer health librarian can probably help you compile a list of good Internet resources.

Taking Your Time

Most health care providers let patients talk for only 22 seconds before taking over the conversation because they are afraid the encounter will last too long if patients are allowed to talk freely. However, research shows that when patients are allowed to speak freely at the beginning of an encounter, they speak for less than 2 minutes. This slight increase in time is certainly worthwhile if it allows patients to give and receive more necessary information, leading to fewer errors and follow-ups.[16]

When you are talking to patients, speak slowly. The concepts you are presenting may be new to them, so they need time to absorb what you say and form questions. Give information in small doses and stop after each to solicit questions and have patients teach back the material (see the next section). Be aware of your body language and tone of voice, which can tell a patient whether you are in a hurry or are ready to take the time to listen to questions and concerns.

Encourage patients to bring a pad and pen along to appointments so they can jot down notes. Note taking

can improve comprehension and retention, and seeing the information in their own words can help patients identify which points need further explanation. It is also helpful to have a family member or trusted friend present during discussions to remember key information and/or take notes for the patient. For patients with low literacy or poor English skills, the elderly, or children, the presence of another person is even more important. In many cases, a family member will be assisting the patient with self-care—whether it is managing medications or maintaining an exercise program—so it is important for him or her to hear the information firsthand as well.

Using Repetitive Education and Teach-Back

Patients remember only about 50% of what they are told, and even that is often incorrect.[17] This makes repetition of information key, because the more you repeat something, the more likely the patient is to retain it. For this to work, all members of the health care team, including physicians, nurses, pharmacists, therapists, nutritionists, and so on, need to reinforce the same message each time they interact with a patient. For instance, if a physician in the emergency department gives a patient a prescription for antibiotics to treat a sinus infection, he or she will instruct the patient to take all of the medication even if symptoms subside. When the nurse gives the patient discharge instructions, he or she will again emphasize the importance of taking the entire prescription no matter how much better the patient feels in the meantime. This point will also be highlighted by the pharmacist who fills the prescription and the label on the bottle.

One of the best ways to determine whether patients have understood the information given to them is to ask them to teach it back to you. After you have explained a diagnosis, treatment plan, or other topic to a patient, ask him or her to repeat this information back to you in his or her own words. Ask open-ended questions such as "What kind of exercise will you do and how often?" rather than questions that require only a "yes" or "no," such as "Do you understand?" If you are teaching a patient how to perform a specific task such as using a home blood pressure cuff or an inhaler, you can use the show-back technique. Here, you ask the patient to demonstrate how he or she will complete the task at home. If a patient cannot explain information or perform a task correctly, try repeating your instructions using simpler language or another method. For instance, some people can remember information only if they see it written down or illustrated. In these cases, you can reinforce your verbal presentation with handouts or instruction sheets that the patient can use as a reference.

Many practitioners are initially resistant to trying teach-back and show-back for fear that it will take too much time. A good strategy for proving the fallacy of this belief is to ask physicians to try these methods with their last patient of the day. This way they do not have to worry about patients backing up in the waiting room, and they can feel more relaxed about making changes to their routine. As they become more comfortable with the process and fine-tune it for their personal style and the information they need to give, they will find that it takes no longer than their previous educational method.

Understanding Media Impact

Anyone who works with patients knows that health information presented by the many available media outlets can strongly influence patients' opinions about conditions and treatments. Consumers are exposed to health warnings on television and in periodicals; direct-to-consumer prescription drug advertising; and mass-media advertisements for health care organizations, medications and supplements, and self-care aids.[18] Many people with fairly high health literacy try to educate themselves about health issues or to even self-diagnose and self-medicate using information from Internet sites and other sources. Those with lower health literacy can be influenced by family members and friends who have seen an article or a program that warned against certain treatments or medicines.

The extent of the impact of mass media is difficult to estimate, but one study looked at women's exposure to newspaper coverage of medical evidence that hormone replacement therapy could have harmful effects. Areas where there was more coverage saw greater declines in the use of such therapy.[19]

It is unlikely that levels of media exposure will decline in the future. Whether it is a patient who thinks he has an incurable disease because he looked up his symptoms on the Internet or someone who wants to know if she can try a prescription drug she saw on television, the members of your health care team need to be prepared for questions based on information from media sources. Because it is nearly impossible to keep up with all the new and experimental treatments and medications being touted, you may not be able to answer some questions immediately. Ask patients where they got their information; you can then review it for validity and applicability.

You should also question patients' flat refusal of suggested treatment options. Although many opinions are formed based on personal and cultural preferences, some people may have come to negative conclusions based on a single news report or their misunderstanding of technical details in an advertisement. Such misconceptions can emphasize the need for providing clear and concise materials of your own.

Making Written Materials Easy to Understand

Health care organizations generate huge amounts of written material: brochures on everything from services offered to health promotion and disease prevention, information on HIPAA and patient rights, history and consent forms, appointment slips/cards, payment notices, discharge and self-care instructions—the list goes on and on. Much of this material is unusable for LEP patients or those who cannot read at (at least) the high school level. This equates to a great deal of wasted time, effort, and money for the organization and a great deal of frustration for the patient.

Revising your existing patient and public materials and establishing policies for creating new ones that your primary audience can read is a logical investment of time and resources. Whether you are trying to ensure that patients know what treatment they are agreeing to, or you are disseminating information on the dangers of obesity, your goals will not be realized unless you can make your message understandable.

Evaluating Materials

When revising one of your existing forms or publications or adopting one from another source, you need to assess its suitability for your patient population. For example, is it written so that patients at all literacy levels can understand it? Mathematical formulas have been used to measure the difficulty level of text has taken place in the United States since the early 1900s.[20] Since then, the practice has become standard across industries to assess both employee and customer materials.

Many readability formulas and scales, including computerized programs, are currently available. Basically, they all use word and sentence length (with multisyllabic words and longer sentences being indicative of greater difficulty) to identify the grade level at which text is written. The main differences between the various formulas are the sample size required and the actual coefficients used in the formula.[21] Given that much of the existing health information for patients is written at the high school or college level, these formulas can help you predict how much you need to simplify the language and writing style of a piece. The following are some of the most common scales that you may choose to employ:

- ➤ Flesch-Kincaid Grade Level
- ➤ Flesch Reading Ease
- ➤ FORCAST
- ➤ Fry Readability Graph
- ➤ Gunning FOG Index (or simply FOG)
- ➤ Lexile Framework for Reading
- ➤ Powers-Sumner-Kearl
- ➤ Simple Measure of Gobbledygook (SMOG)

You can find the actual formulas and explanations of how to use them online at any number of Web sites, including the following:

- ➤ http://www.hsph.harvard.edu
- ➤ http://www.harrymclaughlin.com/SMOG.htm
- ➤ http://www.readabilityformulas.com

The use of formulas is cited fairly regularly in the literature for use with health care–related materials. For example, using SMOG, Gunning FOG, and Flesch-Kincaid Grade Level, researchers at Youngstown State University found that a random sample of online consumer materials provided by national associations for heart disease, cancer, stroke, chronic obstructive pulmonary disease, and diabetes were almost all written above the seventh-grade level and fell into the U.S. Department of Health & Human Services' "difficult" category.[22] A study at the University of Louisville used the Fry Readability Graph to evaluate the reading level of four common depression screening instruments used with postpartum patients, all of which had acceptable second- to fifth-grade levels.[23] Another study at West Virginia University evaluated patient education brochures with the SMOG and Fry methods to determine whether readability improved when medical terminology was deleted; although considerably lower after the deletions, the overall reading levels still ranged from fifth to sixth grade.[24]

In many cases, more than one formula is used because each has a certain range of variability. "It's important to remember to use a formula in context and not rely on it as your sole determinant of readability," notes Lane Stiles, Director of Fairview Press in Minneapolis. "We use a computer program called Readability [Micropower and Light Company] that automatically calculates readability using seven formulas. There is always a range of results. We've learned which formulas tend high and which tend low, and take this into consideration." By using results from this program as a guide, health communications experts at Fairview, which is a division of Fairview Health Systems, have been able to examine various patient forms and brochures and revise them to improve readability (*see* Figure 3-4, page 51).

When using readability formulas you must remember that they have certain limitations. Their emphasis on the number of syllables in a word does not allow for the fact that shorter words (for example, *fetus* or *glucose*) or combination of short words (such as *chest wall pain*) may not be easy for low-literacy patients to understand. Similarly, all multisyllable words are not necessarily difficult; for example, many patients will probably recognize the word *American*.

Figure 3-4. Revision of Patient Information for Better Readability

Dear CPEU Patient:

Admission to the Chest Pain Evaluation Unit (CPEU) initiates a focused assessment of your acute symptoms, which may have included, but are not limited to: chest, neck, shoulder, or arm pain/tightness, or shortness of breath. Multiple tests will be used to determine whether a heart attack (or myocardial infarction in medical terminology) has occurred. Repeat testing over a time frame of several hours is necessary, because heart muscle damage affects changes in blood tests and EKGs that may be delayed from the time of symptom onset. Stress echocardiography will be performed the morning following your admission if there has been no heart muscle injury. The purpose of this test is to observe heart wall motion in response to exercise, which can be a reliable indicator of chest pain due to coronary heart disease.

An Emergency Department staff physician, likely different from your admitting emergency physician, will review test results with you after the stress echocardiogram has been completed and interpreted by a cardiologist. This physician will be much less familiar with your specific case, so please ask any questions you may have about the CPEU process and/or your evaluation during the admitting phase.

Chest pain not due to heart disease may be secondary to many different illnesses. Common examples include musculoskeletal (muscles, ligaments, bones, and joints) chest wall pain, acid-peptic disorders of the stomach and esophagus, and gallbladder disease. Diagnosis of non-heart related symptoms often requires a trial of medication and outpatient reassessment with a primary care physician. Elapsed time assists your follow-up physician to confirm a working diagnosis and recommend additional tests when necessary. Tests to diagnose these potential causes of your symptoms will not be done as part of the CPEU evaluation. If your CPEU evaluation is normal, you will be referred back to a primary care clinic for follow-up, at which time other interventions may be prescribed. If you do not have a primary physician, we will refer you to one. If your CPEU evaluation proves abnormal, an appropriate disposition, which often includes hospital admission, will be arranged.

We hope this information satisfactorily explains the Chest Pain Evaluation Unit concept, mission, and purpose. We wish you well and good health in the future.

Flesch reading ease = 37
Flesch-Kincaid grade level = 13.5
FOG = 16.3
Powers-Sumner-Kearl = 7.4
SMOG = 14.6
FORCAST = 11.0
Fry Graph = 17

A

Welcome to the Chest Pain Evaluation Unit

When you arrive at the Chest Pain Evaluation Unit (CPEU), we may perform a number of tests to see if you've had a heart attack. We may need to repeat these tests over several hours. Feel free to ask questions about your tests or the CPEU at any time.

If you did not have a heart attack, we will do a stress echo (stress echocardiogram) the next morning. This is like an ultrasound test. It lets us observe the motion of your heart wall after you have exercised. It may tell us if you have heart disease.

A doctor in the Emergency Department will explain your test results.

Chest pain can occur for any number of reasons, including:

• bone, joint, muscle or ligament problems

• stomach or esophagus disorders

• gallbladder disease.

If you do not have heart disease, you will need to see your family doctor for further tests. He or she may also try different medicines to see if they affect your symptoms. If you do not have a family doctor, we can suggest one.

If your tests show that you have heart disease, we will discuss your treatment options. We may need to admit you to the hospital.

Flesh Reading Ease = 77
Flesh Grade Level = 5.5
FOG = 7.5
Powers = 5.1
SMOG = 8.3
FORCAST = 9.3
Fry = 7.1

B

Source: Used with permission of Fairview Press.

Fairview Press used an automated program comprising seven readability scales to rate the grade level of this letter given to patients entering Fairview Health Service's Chest Pain Evaluation Unit (A). As shown at the bottom, the text was rated at anywhere from seventh-grade to college level. The revision of the letter uses far less prose, is written in plain English, and is formatted to be less daunting to the eye (B). The reading level range for the revision was between fifth and ninth grade. In each case, the Powers-Summer- Kearl scale gave the lowest level, whereas the others varied.

The results of some formulas, such as Flesch-Kincaid, are significantly affected by punctuation or the addition of headings. Interestingly, punctuation can have even more impact on a scale than how something is written. "At a conference on health literacy, I once demonstrated that the readability of a document would remain the same even if you reversed the words in every sentence, as long as you used the same punctuation," recalls Stiles. "If we were to judge readability solely in terms of readability formulas, we'd risk giving our patients absolute gobbledygook, which, unfortunately, we sometimes do."

Although readability formulas are good tools for determining how well your material meets the functional literacy level of your audience, other factors are just as important. Stiles recommends that organizations use health communications specialists to review forms and publications for suitability of purpose, audience, relevance, scope, flow and coherence, formatting, use of graphics, and cultural appropriateness. "It's a lot harder to make documents readable than people think," he says. "Many of us are seriously blinded by our jargon, by the ways we've been formally trained to structure knowledge. Instead of focusing on key messages—what patients need to know—we overwhelm them with anatomy, physiology, and other types of 'nice to know' information."

Developing Reader-Friendly Materials

After you have assessed your existing forms and brochures, you will need some guidelines to follow when revising them; these same guidelines can be applied to any new materials you create. The following are some considerations about low-literacy readers to keep in mind as you formulate your strategies[21]:

➤ They tend to think in concrete, immediate terms rather than in abstract concepts or for the long run.

➤ They accept information at face value and interpret instructions and graphics literally.

➤ They do not know how to apply new information to their existing knowledge.

➤ Because they tend to read slowly and skip words they find too difficult, they often do not grasp meaning or context. They also tend to lose interest quickly.

➤ When faced with supporting details, they often lose track of the main message.

Your goal is to design materials that compensate for these weaknesses. Most of the strategies you are likely to use can be divided into the categories of content, writing style, format, and use of graphics. Your guidelines should include criteria for all of these elements.

If your organization is large, and different departments develop their own written pieces, be sure that all authors receive a copy of your guidelines so the quality of materials is uniform. When consistency among different areas and messages is a problem, it can help to have a central committee or group that reviews all materials before they are printed.

Content

You can save a great deal of time and effort if you do some planning before you ever write a word. Your first step is to decide what the objective of the material is, who it is meant for, and how it will be used. Use the worksheet in Figure 3-5 (page 53) to help you answer these questions and organize your writing efforts.

When you have a clear picture of the final piece, you can start to gather your content information. Because many readers have a short attention span, include only information that is essential for meeting your stated goal; forms should also ask only for information that is absolutely necessary so patients do not feel overwhelmed. Limit the length of the piece based on what you can reasonably expect the reader to learn at one time. Focus on providing instructions for and examples of desired behavior rather than medical facts. Finally, make sure that any examples you use are appropriate to the demographics, language, and experience of your audience.[25]

Writing Style

Remember that you are writing for laypeople who may have very low literacy and/or English skills, not a journal for health care professionals. Formal, third-person narrative can be boring and off-putting, so consider using a conversational tone and writing in the active voice. Replace all medical, legal, or complicated words with plain language, and if you must use a specialized term, explain it in simple words.[25] You may find online plain-language glossaries, such as those for asthma, arthritis, and lupus on Harvard School of Public Health's Web site (http://www.hsph.harvard.edu/healthliteracy/innovative.html), helpful in explaining complex ideas. Write for a fifth-grade level or lower to help make the material clear to everyone. Generalizations such as *many* or *normal* mean nothing to low-literacy readers, so use specific terms and parameters such as "5 to 10" or "98.6°F."

Use simple sentence structure and keep each paragraph short and focused on only one topic. When you present new information or ideas, give the context first[25]; for example, "To spot any early signs of breast cancer [*context*], you need to have a test called a mammogram once a year [*information*]."

State your objective clearly at the beginning of the piece and then break up material into manageable chunks. Use headings to set off new ideas and alert readers to key messages. Review those key messages at the end of a short piece or periodically throughout a

Figure 3-5. Planning Worksheet for Written Materials

What Are Our Goals?

Do we want this piece to inform (about diseases, treatments, etc.), model new behaviors, motivate readers to do (or not do) something? _____

_____

What do we want the reader's response to be? _____

_____

If this is a form, are we collecting or giving information (for example, medical history, versus informed consent form)?

_____

_____

Who Is Our Target Audience?

Age group _____

Gender _____

Ethnicity _____

Income level _____

Education level _____

Health literacy level _____

Cultural preferences and religious beliefs that may affect attitudes toward this topic _____

Level of experience with the health care system _____

Health status (physical and psychological) _____

How Will We Use This Piece?

Will the reader use this piece alone or as part of an encounter with a health care professional?

_____

Is this a stand-alone product, or is it part of a series? _____

Where and when will we distribute it? _____

For forms, is the user meant to fill this out alone or with the help of staff? _____

Do similar forms exist in other departments (for example, informed consent for surgery, diagnostic services, nuclear medicine)? _____

If so, is there any redundancy that can be removed? _____

If the goal of this form is to gather information, what will that information be used for (for example, the care process, process improvement)? _____

Sources: Doak L.G., Doak C.C. (eds.): *Pfizer Principles for Clear Health Communication,* 2nd ed. Pfizer, Inc., 2004. http://www.pfizerhealthliteracy.com/pdf/PfizerPrinciples.pdf (accessed Dec. 30, 2008); Doak C.C., Doak L.G., Root J.H.: *Teaching Patients with Low Literacy Skills,* 2nd ed. Philadelphia: J. B. Lippincott Company, 1996; National Cancer Institute: *Clear & Simple: Developing Effective Print Materials for Low-Literate Readers.* http://www.nci.nih.gov/cancerinformation/clearandsimple (accessed Dec. 30, 2008).

Using these questions can allow you to structure your writing efforts more efficiently. You probably already have a great deal of this information. (See the section on data collection in Chapter 2 (pages 33–34) and "Understanding the Patient's Perspective" on page 38 in this chapter.)

longer piece to help readers remember them. Another way to stimulate long-term memory is to ask readers to solve problems, make choices, or perform a task based on the information given. The more interactive you can make the material, the better.[25]

Some of these principles also apply when you are working with forms. State exactly what you want the reader to do in each section—check boxes, fill in blanks, circle applicable items, and so on. Use plain language; for example, on a medical history form, you might substitute *high blood pressure* for *hypertension* and *low blood sugar* for *hypoglycemia*.

Forms that pertain to financial information and insurance can tax the understanding of any patient, including college graduates. Most are written with legal requirements rather than readability in mind, and organizations often try to squeeze as much information as possible onto one sheet. The two versions of the payment form in Figure 3-6 (page 55) illustrate how revising both language and formatting can help patients comprehend what is required of them financially and make an informed choice to accept or decline services.

Format

With the extensive capabilities of today's software, the temptation to dress up your materials with decorative fonts and borders or wrap text around graphics can be strong. Resist it. What looks artistic to you can make a piece look intimidating to readers with low literacy. Here is a list of recommendations to help you keep to a reader-friendly format[21,25,26]:

➤ Use 12-point (or larger) serif type for text and do not use more than two fonts.

➤ Do not use all capital letters, italics, or reverse type, all of which are difficult to read. Use boldface for keywords or emphasis only.

➤ Surround text with plenty of white space so pages do not appear cluttered or dense.

➤ Use "cueing devices"—arrows, boxes, and so on—to direct readers' attention to specific points.

➤ Keep line length to between 30 and 50 characters and spaces.

➤ Leave the right margin jagged to avoid hyphen-ating words at the ends of lines.

➤ Use matte or low-gloss paper and make sure there is a high contrast between the type and your chosen paper.

➤ Use color sparingly to add emphasis.

➤ Do not use lists longer than three to five items. If you have a longer list, break up items into smaller groups with subheadings to separate them.

➤ Place graphics as close as possible to the corresponding text.

If you are designing a form, you should follow most of the same rules. Type needs to be easy to read, and you should leave white space between items and around the margins so readers will see each item. When asking for written responses, allow enough room for those responses. Many forms leave only a small line for each answer, even when descriptive narrative is requested; patients often skip these items.

Use of Graphics

As with face-to-face communication, understanding and retention can be heightened with the correct use of visual aids—in this case, photos or drawings. And as with text formatting, there is a great temptation to use graphics to make a piece "look nice." Remember that low-level readers take pictures literally, so extraneous material will only confuse them. If you choose to include graphics in your product, use only those that are directly linked to and help explain the text. Each picture should have an explanatory caption. If you use graphs or charts, keep them simple and explain clearly how readers should use them or what point from the text they illustrate.[25]

Keep pictures simple and focused on the main theme or action; avoid cluttered backgrounds in photos and overly detailed diagrams. Whether you use photos or drawings, the actions should be depicted realistically. For example, if you are using a drawing instead of a photo to show patients how to give themselves injections, be sure that the positioning of hands and injection sites is anatomically feasible (a rough draft of one organization's brochure on insulin administration included a drawing of a man injecting himself in the back in a way that would be impossible for any normal adult). If you are

Figure 3-6. Improvement of a Payment Notification Form

____ Account Number

FAIRVIEW

Non-Emergent Patient Notification Form

Patient Name: ____

Medical Record Number: ____

Date of Service: ____

Procedures/Services:
- ❑ Non- Emergent Visit: 80% deposit required of estimated charges.

  Estimated Charges: ____ Deposit for Facility Fees: ____
- ❑ Known Procedures/Services: ____

Read each condition carefully. Please mark the one situation that best fits your preference for payment:

____ I understand Fairview Health Systems may not or does not have a participation contract with my health plan and that I may be considered self-pay. My signature on this form indicates that I am financially liable for the services being provided.

____ The Medicare system shows another insurance as primary. Medicare is primary.
I (member) will contact Medicare to inform them of the change.

____ I have health insurance, but I do not wish to have my health plan billed or notified. I do not wish to be considered a member of my health plan for the above services. My signature on this form indicates that I am financially liable for the services being provided.

____ I am a member in the following health plan and do not have an authorized referral for the service(s) listed above or those services are determined to be non-covered by my insurance plan. My signature on this form indicates that I may be financially liable for the services being provided.

- ☐ Blue Cross
- ☐ Health Partners
- ☐ Medica
- ☐ Metropolitan Health Plan
- ☐ U Care
- ☐ Preferred One
- ☐ Other: ____

____ I understand that I do not have health insurance and I am considered self-pay. My signature on this form indicates that I am financially liable for the services being provided.

____ Patient refuses to sign this form.

Patient Signature ____ Date ____

Responsible Party Signature ____ Date ____

Refusal of Service for Non-Emergent Visits:
My provider has explained the estimated cost of the care described above. I understand that I can decide whether or not to have the service(s) listed above. I do NOT want to have the services listed above, because I do not want to pay for the service(s) myself.

Patient Signature ____ Date ____

Responsible Party Signature ____ Date ____

Original – Health Information Management Copy Yellow – Patient / Authorized Person Copy

A

Patient name: ____

Medical record number: ____

Date of service: ____

Patient Identification Label

Notice of Payment for Non-Emergency Care

Known services: ____

- ❑ If you will pay for these services yourself, we refer to you as "self-pay."
  - You will need to pay a deposit before we provide these services.
    Your deposit will be: $____. This is 80% of the estimated total charge: $____.
  - We may use a screening program to see if you qualify for medical assistance or Fairview's community care program. These programs may help pay for your care.

Preferred method of payment: Check the correct box below.
(You may need to call your health plan. Ask if they have a contract with Fairview Health Services.)

- ❑ Fairview may not—or does not—have a contract with my health plan. **If it does not, I agree to pay for all services provided.**
- ❑ Fairview has a contract with my health plan. I do **not** want Fairview to bill my health plan or inform it of services I receive. **I agree to pay for all services provided.**
- ❑ I have one of the health plans listed below *(check one)*. I am told that my plan will not pay for the above services **or** I do not have an authorized referral for these services. (A referral is written approval from your family doctor or clinic.) **I may need to pay for the services provided. Or I may be asked to pay a larger part of the total bill.**
  - ❑ Blue Cross ❑ Medica ❑ U Care ❑ Metropolitan Health Plan (MHP)
  - ❑ Health Partners ❑ Preferred One ❑ Other: ____
- ❑ I do not have health insurance. **I agree to pay for all services provided.**
- ❑ I am on Medicare. I am told that Medicare lists another health plan as the primary payer (the first payer to be billed for my services). This is not correct. Medicare is the primary payer. **I will contact Medicare to inform them of the change.**
- ❑ I refuse to sign this form.

Patient signature: ____ Date: ____

Responsible party's signature: ____ Date: ____

Refusal of service:
I do **not** want to have the services listed above, because I do not want to pay for them myself.

Patient signature: ____ Date: ____

Responsible party's signature: ____ Date: ____

Fairview Health Services NOTICE OF PAYMENT FOR NON-EMERGENCY CARE

476539 – REV 08/08 *White – CBO Scanner 400 Stinson* *Yellow/Copy – Patient* *Pink/Copy – Medical Records* Page 1 of 1 C/D4a

B

Source: Used with permission of Fairview Press.

Even the title of the original version of this form was unclear and did not tell patients the point of filling it out (A). Although the patient only needed to check off appropriate statements, those statements were written at a level that many would find difficult to understand. The combination of boxes and blank lines also can be confusing. The revised form (B) uses clear language, highlights the most important points in bold type, and is formatted consistently in lists with check boxes.

gearing a piece toward a specific ethnic or cultural group, people from that group should be represented in the supporting photos and drawings.[25,27]

Although you can have photos taken or drawings created specifically for your piece, this option can be costly. In many cases, you may be able to download graphics from online resources at little or no cost. For example, pictograms that you can insert in patient education materials are available free on the U.S. Pharmacopeia Web site (http://www.usp.org). The set comprises 80 different graphic symbols depicting various instructions for medication use (*see* Figure 3-7, page 56) that can be printed out separately as reminders to be posted in the home, dropped into preprinted schedules and instruction sheets, or included in brochures.

Getting Patient Feedback

There are distinct advantages to soliciting patient input during all stages of material development. As mentioned earlier, patients feel empowered when you ask for and use their opinions. The sense of ownership that is generated makes it more likely that they will use the final product and encourage others to do so as well.

Figure 3-7. Examples of U.S. Pharmacopeia Pictograms

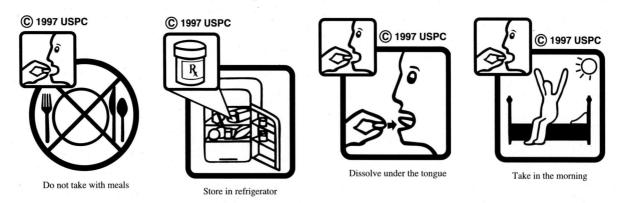

Do not take with meals   Store in refrigerator   Dissolve under the tongue   Take in the morning

Source: © The United States Pharmacopeial Convention. Used with permission.

You can use pictograms like the ones shown here to complement all types of patient education materials. The full set of 80 symbols was developed by the U.S. Pharmacopeia.

Obtaining patients' views up front can also help you create a piece that is more appropriate for your target audience than it would be otherwise.[28,29] For example, you might ask patients to look at different graphics that are being considered for a new brochure. As potential readers, they can tell you which ones they consider helpful and attractive; they may also suggest a picture that you have not thought of.

Patients are also good reviewers during the draft and pilot-testing stages. You may ask them to evaluate the entire product or individual elements such as readability, usefulness of content, or design.

There are different ways of getting user input. Your organization may have a patient advisory council or public members on your board of directors. Although they can apply their personal experiences to any materials you show them, they are more likely to have higher levels of health literacy. This means they may not be able to judge whether something is understandable for the elderly, LEP patients, and other high-risk populations. You may choose to convene focus groups, which can bring together members of your target audience but can also prove to be both time-consuming and labor-intensive to set up and prepare for.

Another alternative is the informal interview, men-

tioned earlier in this chapter, which staff members can conduct during "downtimes" in the care process. Unless they are in pain, most people welcome a distraction while they are waiting to see a physician or therapist, receive test results, or pick up a prescription. Home health nurses might take a few extra minutes at the end of each home visit to ask patients or families for input on materials, and long term care staff may talk to family members who are waiting while residents are being bathed or receiving treatment. You may find it helpful to work out a script in advance for all interviewers to use; the suggestions for asking people to participate in health literacy testing (*see* "Widely Used Tests" on page 27 in Chapter 2) can be adapted to fit information gathering or pilot testing. The same rules apply, as follows:

➤ Be honest and clear about what you are doing.

➤ Ask for their help.

➤ Do not make people feel as though they have been singled out for some negative reason (such as low literacy or low income).

➤ Respect refusals and move on to the next person.

Making Translations Available

You need to have print materials, particularly consent forms, available in all the languages commonly spoken by your patient populations. Although this may seem like an overwhelming task, your organization is responsible for making sure that information is pre-

Figure 3-8. Confusing Prescription Warning Labels

Are These Clear?

 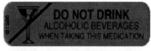 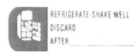

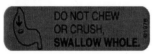 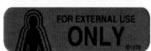 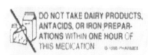

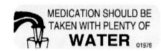 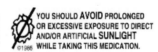 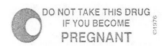

All short and seemingly simple

Source: Terry C. Davis. Used with permission.

Icons, colors, and text used on warning labels such as these can cause more confusion than they alleviate. Patients with poor literacy or English skills may formulate all types of interpretations. For example, "Take with food" can be interpreted as "Don't take food." The label specifying "For external use only" may turn into "Use extreme caution in how you take it" or "Take only if you need it" when the patient reads it.

sented to patients in ways they can understand, and this refers to preferred language as well as reading level. Whenever print pieces are revised or new ones created, translations should be revised or created as well.

Quality control of translated material can be difficult, so always use a professional translator or service. Remember that translators can work only with the material they are given, so if the language level in your original piece is too high, the level of the translations will be as well. This is another stage at which patient feedback can be invaluable. Patients with limited or no English skills can let you know whether a translation is readable, whether specific terms have the same meaning in different cultural contexts, and whether the product is useful.

Improving Medication Instructions and Labels

Medication errors may be the most common type of

adverse event across all health care settings. As care continues to shift from inpatient to outpatient settings, patients are assuming more responsibility for self-administering medications. Add to this complications such as drug regimens that are complex and require several medications to be taken at specific times, or older adults who have multiple medications that are prescribed by several practitioners and filled by both local and mail-order pharmacies. The threat to patient safety is significant, even for those who have relatively high health literacy. Much of the problem is due to poor verbal and written communication between patients and providers. Many patients find it difficult to comprehend the instructions on handouts and prescription bottles, let alone decipher the name of the drug or the dense clinical information included as a separate insert.

Several studies have examined patient difficulties in interpreting prescription drug labels.[30–33] The most fre-

Figure 3-9. Cantonese Version of a Visual Medication Schedule

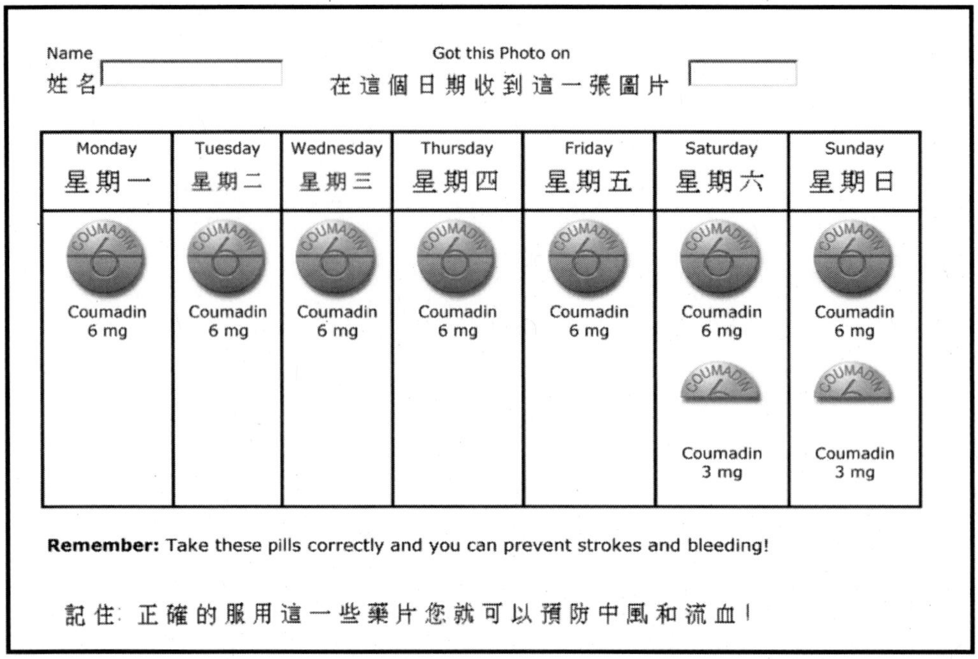

Source: Machtinger E.L., et al.: A visual medication schedule to improve anticoagulation control: A randomized, controlled trial. *Jt Comm J Qual Patient Saf* 33:625–633, Oct. 2007.

This example of a computer-generated schedule has digitized color images of the pills (Coumadin) the individual patient should take on a weekly basis. Developed to improve patient-provider communication about anticoagulant care, this one-page schedule can be generated in English alone or with Spanish or Cantonese translations. It can be used in conjunction with counseling provided by a pharmacist, cardiologist, or other health professional.

quent misunderstandings were associated with dosage amount and frequency, and although such problems were most common in patients with low literacy, those with adequate literacy levels also had trouble. The causes of misunderstandings included the following:

➤ Instructions given in multiple steps instead of a single step were difficult for most people to follow.

➤ Patients with good reading skills tended to think that instructions were simple and read them quickly, whereas those with poor reading skills could not understand many of the words when text was written at the high school level or higher. In each case, comprehension suffered.

➤ Dosing instructions that were written in imprecise terms, such as "Take two capsules by mouth twice daily," forced patients to figure out the appropriate dosing times. They also became confused about how many pills to take.

➤ Prescription labels emphasized information that was important to the pharmacy and prescriber rather than the patient, such as the prescription order number, the generic and brand names of the drug, and the refill date.

➤ Pamphlets and instructions were written at high school or higher levels and included a great deal of information that patients did not need or use.

➤ Patients sometimes ignored or misinterpreted the special warning labels on the bottle, finding the icons, colors, and/or text unclear (*see* Figure 3-8, page 57). Researchers have suggested several ways to improve labeling and instructions for medications[30–35]:

➤ Write instructions for prescription labels as clearly and concisely as possible, using simple wording and Arabic numerals instead of words for all numbers. For example, "Take 2 tablets at breakfast and 2 tablets at dinner" is clearer than "Take two tablets every 12 hours."

Using *morning* and *evening* are also clear and allow patients to fit the doses into their schedules. With complex regimens that depend on doses of several medications being taken at specific times, list those times on the label (for example, "Take 1 capsule at 8 A.M. and 2 capsules at 4:30 P.M.").

➤ Reorganize labels to minimize "distracters" such as the pharmacy logo and other information that is directed at providers instead of patients. Use highlighting, boldface, and/or large type for dosing instructions, warnings, and indications, and try to arrange labels so they do not overlap or obscure important text.

➤ The importance of teach-back has already been discussed, but it is particularly vital in talking with patients about medications. Even when they read back a label correctly, some people may not be able to count out the correct number of pills or may use a tablespoon instead of the required teaspoon. Many clinics, hospitals, and physician offices are trying to provide instruction sheets for patients to help them understand and remember how and when to take their medications. Limit the information in such materials to what patients actually need to know (including the name of the drug, when and how to take it, indications of an adverse reaction, and who to contact for help). Use plain language and other principles already described for creating print pieces. For example, handouts that use graphics, such as the medication schedule shown in Figure 3-9 (*see* page 58), can make it easier for patients to keep track of what they should be taking and when.

➤ When labels or instructions are translated into different languages, the text and icons must be translated correctly and consistently, and cultural differences must be taken into account.

➤ Consumers, particularly those with low literacy, should be actively involved in developing new labels, handouts, and educational materials to ensure that the icons, words, and formatting are clear and useful to everyone.

Making Your Web Site More User Friendly

Although not a print medium, a Web site can be the first exposure patients have to your organization, and many of the same rules you use for other written materials can be applied to the information you provide online. For example, text should use plain language and the active voice, and difficult terms should be explained (only in this case, you can link such words to an online glossary). You will also want to break information into short, manageable sections and use only images that directly apply to the text. If many of your patients have limited English skills, you will need to make translations of the site text available in the prevalent languages of your community. Make backgrounds plain, and put dark type on a light background rather than using light on dark or strong colors for both type and background.

There are any number of online and local professional services available to evaluate your Web site and make recommendations, but the following are a few basic suggestions to get you started[36]:

➤ If you use video or audio clips, make segments short to avoid long download times on older systems.

➤ Make your site as easy to navigate as possible. Label links carefully and organize the site so users can move from page to page in a logical sequence.

➤ Use the same symbols and icons throughout the site and use the same navigation buttons in the same place on each page. Use the same basic design for each page.

➤ Avoid pull-down menus whenever possible.

➤ Make sure that your organization's name, address, telephone number, and e-mail address are displayed prominently on your home page so users can contact you in whatever way they find easiest.

Remember that, as with all your other educational materials, you create a Web site for your patients and community. If you try to design your site for those with low levels of literacy, English proficiency, and computer knowledge, you will make it easier for everyone to use.

Many of the interventions suggested in this chapter should be applicable or adaptable to your organization and patients. Chapter 4 presents real-world case studies that show how a variety of organizations used the methods described here, as well as their own techniques, to raise their populations' health literacy levels and to improve communication of information.

References

1. Office of Disease Prevention and Health Promotion, U.S. Department of Health & Human Services: *Health Communication Activities: Sample Action Plan to Improve Health Literacy.* http://www.health.gov/communication/literacy/sampleplan.htm (accessed Feb. 15, 2009).

2. Nelson J.C., Schwartzberg J.G., Vergara K.C.: The public's and the patient's right to know: AMA commentary on "Public Health in America: An Ethical Imperative." *Am J Prev Med* 28(3):325–326, 2005.

3. Nielsen-Bohlman L.N., Panzer A.M., Kindig D.A. (eds.): *Health Literacy: A Prescription to End Confusion.* Washington, DC: National Academies Press, 2004.

4. The Joint Commission: *"What Did the Doctor Say?" Improving Health Literacy to Protect Patient Safety* (white paper). Oakbrook Terrace, IL: 2007.

5. Harper W., Cook S., Makoul G.: Teaching medical students about health literacy: 2 Chicago initiatives. *Am J Health Behav* 31(suppl. 1):S111–S114, 2007.

6. Rudd R.E.: The patient perspective: Introduction. In Schwartzberg J.G., VanGeest J.B., Wang C.C. (eds.): *Understanding Health Literacy: Implications for Medicine and Public Health.* Chicago: American Medical Association, 2005, p. 41.

7. Joint Commission Resources: Cultural and linguistic issues in the informed consent process. *The Joint Commission: The Source* 5:3–4, Jul. 2007.

8. Ngo-Metzger Q., et al.: *Cultural Competency and Quality of Care: Obtaining the Patient's Perspective.* Commonwealth Fund, Oct. 2006. http://www.cmwf.org/usr_doc/Ngo-Metzger_cultcompqualitycareobtainpatientperspect_963.pdf (accessed Dec. 30, 2008).

9. Divi C., et al.: Language proficiency and adverse events in US hospitals: A pilot study. *Int J Qual Health Care* 19(2):60–67, 2007.

10. Ngo-Metzger Q., et al.: Providing high-quality care for limited English proficient patients: The importance of language concordance and interpreter use. *J Gen Intern Med* 22(suppl. 2):324–330, 2007.

11. Joint Commission Resources: Promoting effective communication—Language access services in health care. *Jt Comm Perspect* 28:8–11, Feb. 2008.

12. Schyve P.M.: Language differences as a barrier to quality and safety in health care: The Joint Commission perspective. *J Gen Intern Med* 22(suppl. 2):360–361, 2007.

13. Kallail K.J.: Communicating with patients at risk for low health literacy. *Kansas Journal of Medicine* 1(1):22–26, 2007.

14. Weiss B.D.: *Health Literacy and Patient Safety: Help Patients Understand. Manual for Clinicians,* 2nd ed. Chicago: American Medical Association Foundation and American Medical Association, 2007.

15. Brey R.A., Clark S.E., Wantz M.S.: Enhancing health literacy through accessing health information, products, and services: An exercise for children and adolescents. *J Sch Health* 77:640–644, Nov. 2007.

16. Partnership for Clear Health Communication at the National Patient Safety Foundation: *What Can Providers Do?* http://www.npsf.org/askme3/PCHC/what_can_provid.php (accessed Dec. 30, 2008).

17. DeWalt D.A.: Low health literacy: Epidemiology and interventions. *N C Med J* 68:327–330, Sep.–Oct. 2007.

18. Paasche-Orlow M.K., et al.: How health care systems can begin to address the challenge of limited literacy. *J Gen Intern Med* 21:884–887, 2006.

19. Haas J.S., et al.: Average household exposure to newspaper coverage about the harmful effects of hormone therapy and population-based declines in hormone therapy use. *J Gen Intern Med* 22:68–73, 2007.

20. Scott B.: *The History and Development of Readability Formulas.* http://www.readabilityformulas.com/articles/history-and-development-of-readability-formulas.php (accessed Dec. 30, 2008).

21. Doak C.C., Doak L., Root J.H.: *Teaching Patients with Low Literacy Skills,* 2nd ed. Philadelphia: J. B. Lippincott Company, 1996.

22. Walsh T.M., Volsko T.A.: Readability assessment of Internet-based consumer health information. *Respir Care* 53:1310–1315, Oct. 2008.

23. Logsdon M.C., Hutti M.H.: Readability: An important issue impacting healthcare for women with postpartum depression. *MCN Am J Matern Child Nurs* 31:350–355, Nov.–Dec. 2006.

24. Sand-Jecklin K.: The impact of medical terminology on readability of patient education materials. *J Community Health Nurs* 24(2):119–129, 2007.

25. Doak L.G., Doak C.C. (eds.): *Pfizer Principles for Clear Health Communication,* 2nd ed. Pfizer Inc., 2004. http://www.pfizerhealthliteracy.com/pdf/PfizerPrinciples.pdf (accessed Dec. 30, 2008).

26. Rudd R.E.: *How to Create and Assess Print Materials.* Harvard School of Public Health: Health Literacy Studies, 2005. http://www.hsph.harvard.edu/healthliteracy/materials.html (accessed Dec. 30, 2008).

27. Monachos C.L.: Assessing and addressing low health literacy among surgical outpatients. *AORN J* 86:373–383, Sep. 2007.

28. Kreps G.L., Sparks L.: Meeting the health literacy needs of immigrant populations. *Patient Educ Couns* 71:328–332, 2008.

29. Shaw S.J., et al.: The role of culture in health literacy and chronic disease screening and management. *J Immigr Minor Health,* Apr. 1, 2008. [E-pub].

30. Davis T.C., et al.: Low literacy impairs comprehension of prescription drug warning labels. *J Gen Intern Med* 21:847–851, 2006.

31. Wolf M.S., et al.: Misunderstanding of prescription drug warning labels among patients with low literacy. *Am J Health Syst Pharm* 63:1048–1055, Jun. 1, 2006.

32. Wolf M.S., et al.: To err is human: Patient misinterpretations of prescription drug label instructions. *Patient Education and Counseling* 67:293–300, 2007.

33. Davis T.C., et al.: Literacy and misunderstanding prescription drug labels. *Ann Intern Med* 145(12):887–894, Dec. 19, 2006.

34. Wolf M.S., Bailey S.C.: Improving prescription drug labeling. *N C Med J* 68(5):340–342, Sep./Oct. 2007.

35. Machtinger E.L., et al.: A visual medication schedule to improve anticoagulation control: A randomized, controlled trial. *Jt Comm J Qual Patient Saf* 33:625–633, Oct. 2007.

36. National Institute on Aging and National Library of Medicine: *Making Your Web Site Senior Friendly: A Checklist.* http://www.nlm.nih.gov/pubs/checklist.pdf (accessed Dec. 30, 2008).

CHAPTER 4
CASE STUDIES

The case studies in this chapter address many of the solutions and suggestions described in Chapter 3. Topics range from the development of a health literacy curriculum for medical schools, to the creation of teaching aids for specific populations, to improving language services, to establishing health literacy programs for health systems and individual states. You will find that many of these organizations have faced the same types of challenges you do in finding ways to improve their patients' health literacy, regardless of service type or size.

CASE STUDY: BRONSON HEALTHCARE GROUP

Because health literacy affects so many aspects of care quality and safety, health care organizations can see it as a vital part of an overall push for better performance. Bronson Healthcare Group serves the city of Kalamazoo and the surrounding areas in southwest Michigan and northern Indiana. The system includes three hospitals, including Bronson Methodist Hospital, its 380-bed flagship facility; an outpatient center; home health care; and physician practices. Recipient of the 2005 Malcolm Baldrige National Quality Award, Bronson has closely linked its strategic plan to the Institute of Medicine's (IOM's) six quality aims of (1) safety, (2) patient centeredness, (3) effectiveness, (4) efficiency, (5) equity, and (6) timeliness. The aim of patient centeredness works with the key strategies of clinical excellence and customer service excellence, and several of these strategies have been related to health literacy. They include a health literacy task force, a campaign to encourage patients and families to ask questions and be actively involved with their care, and an information center that helps patients find reliable health information in formats they can understand.

Focusing on Health Literacy

Bronson has identified poor health literacy as a concern based on the low education levels in some of its service areas. "People always say you can't equate education with literacy, but if someone hasn't completed high school, there's a fair chance that their reading level is lower than you would expect," notes Marge Kars, M.L.S., A.H.I.P., manager of Bronson's Health Sciences Library and Bronson HealthAnswers. Data from the National Institute for Literacy's 1998 *The State of Literacy in America* (which provides tables estimating the literacy level of populations by state, city, and county) and the 2003 National Adult Literacy Survey helped staff calculate the probable percentages of communities that were at risk for low reading literacy.

Potential problems for non-English-speaking populations were also recognized. Kalamazoo is home to two

colleges and Western Michigan University, so Bronson facilities may serve patients with a wide range of languages and backgrounds when classes are in session. Although its year-round Hispanic population is small (about 3%), the health care needs of this group are significant.

In 2003 Bronson formed its Health Literacy Task Force with the following goals:

➤ To provide high-quality, audience-appropriate health information for specific health problems and health-related decisions

➤ To train health care professionals and support staff in the use of communication tools to better support the individual health information needs of patients and their families

The task force was made up of clinical and support staff—including representatives from nursing, pharmacy, education, and finance—from across the system's hospitals and physician practices.

For six months, the task force met to discuss health literacy issues, evaluate patient forms, and plan for staff training on nursing units and in physician practices. When some of the original members left the task force, staff from the Education Services Department became responsible for staff training. The Forms Committee, which was charged with reviewing all clinical and patient forms, incorporated easy-reading guidelines for readability into its review process. Both groups report directly to Bronson's Continuum of Care Committee, which comprises administrative staff, nurses, physicians, and support staff such as information technology representatives. This group is dedicated to making sure patients have a seamless care experience and includes health literacy in its planning for care and discharge processes.

Simplifying Written Materials

One of the first projects addressed by the task force and subsequent committees was improving the readabil-

Figure 4-1. Survey Form for Readability of Written Materials

Patient Feedback Survey
Bronson Patient and Family Education Committee

Please rate the following statements about the document you just read on a scale of 1 to 5, with 1 being **strongly disagree** to 5 being **strongly agree.**

		Strongly Disagree	Somewhat Disagree	Neutral	Somewhat Agree	Strongly Agree
1.	The title of the pamphlet/ booklet reflects its contents.	1	2	3	4	5
2.	The information is easy to understand.	1	2	3	4	5
3.	The medical words are explained.	1	2	3	4	5
4.	The sentences are short.	1	2	3	4	5
5.	The print is large enough to read.	1	2	3	4	5
6.	The information is useful.	1	2	3	4	5
7.	The diagrams or drawings are easy to understand.	1	2	3	4	5

8. Would you recommend this material to a family member or friend who is going through the same experience?
   ___Yes   ___No

9. Your overall evaluation of this material:
   ___Poor   __Fair   __Average   __Good   __Outstanding

10 I am (please check):
   ❑ A patient
   ❑ A patient's family member
   ❑ A patient's friend
   ❑ Other

Additional comments:

_____

_____

_____

_____

_____

_____

Thank you for your help.

Source: Used with permission from Bronson Healthcare Group.

This survey is given to patient volunteers who review Bronson's forms and educational brochures for usefulness and readability.

ity of forms and educational materials used by patients and families. Staff originally determined that an eighth-grade reading level would make information understandable to most patients; this was later lowered to a sixth-grade reading level, and staff are now working to rewrite consent forms at the fifth-grade level. All new and revised forms must follow the system's guidelines for readability, including being written in the active voice, using everyday language and short sentences, and having easy-to-read formatting with lots of white space. Commonly used forms are translated into Spanish.

Two staff members meet biweekly to look at forms that require revision. The first to be addressed were the consent for operation and treatment, admission and registration forms, and discharge instructions. Community volunteers from the system's Patient and Family Advisory Council are asked to look at forms and complete a survey (*see* Figure 4-1, page 63) regarding their readability and usefulness to patients. "We ask them to look at font size, whether the title reflects the content of the brochure, whether it's easy to understand, whether we've explained the medical words, whether the information was useful, whether they would recommend the brochure to family members, and so on," explains Kars. "We don't want people who are familiar with the terminology, test, or condition to review the material. They would only say, 'I get it,' or, 'This is much too easy.' So we continue to use volunteers."

Some departments found it difficult to comply with the new guidelines while keeping forms to their traditional length. For example, staff in registration preferred to give patients one piece of paper to sign, which sometimes meant that an informed consent form was printed in very small type. Staff from the Forms Committee explained that 12-point type and a format that includes plenty of white space is the standard for all Bronson forms. According to Kars, "One page is not our standard. Our standard is to put the information into however many pages it takes so the patient can read it easily."

Training Staff

The Health Literacy Task Force's original aims were to look at written materials, work with the community,

and educate staff. The focus for the first year was primarily on revision and translation of forms, but in 2004 the push for staff training in health literacy grew. Bronson purchased the American Medical Association (AMA) Foundation video *Helping Your Patients Understand* and made it a part of staff orientation throughout Bronson Healthcare Group.

Recognizing that low general and health literacy isn't limited to patients, Bronson began looking at the needs of its 5,000 employees. "Everyone is supposed to be at least a high school graduate, but that doesn't mean they all read at the high school level," says Kars. "There are people who frequently don't read at the levels you would expect or that they need." With this in mind, leaders created a partnership with a community adult education agency to provide classes in mathematics, English as a second language, and reading for employees. Sessions are confidential and take place at work, so individuals can upgrade their skills; a few have even gone on to get their general equivalency diplomas.

Communication techniques such as teach-back and Ask Me 3™ have been taught to throughout the system, and teach-back is now a clinical assignment for all new nurses coming into the organization. After orientation, they work one-on-one with a mentor for a few months and are given various assignments to complete. The mentor models the practice of teach-back, then the nurses use it on their own. This practice is being expanded to include all respiratory therapists and other allied health staff, and teach-back will be included as a competency on their performance evaluations.

The most common complaint staff have about using teach-back is that they don't have time. As Kars points out, it helps to present this technique as a short-term investment with long-term benefits: "It's sometimes difficult to explain to people that at the beginning it might take longer, but they'll be amazed that it really doesn't take as long as they think it will, and they're giving the information in a way that the patient can understand. This means the patient isn't going to come back to the office or be readmitted to the hospital because he didn't take his medication, or she's going to show up for her test prepared so it doesn't have to be rescheduled."

In 2008 Bronson's Customer Service Department established a systemwide program called Teaming Up for Patients and Family-Centered Care, which is mandatory for all employees and clinical staff. Part of the four-hour class is dedicated to building relationships among members of the care team. There is also a section on communication, including tools and strategies for talking to patients, giving and receiving feedback, and handing off patients between settings. To give participants a visual aid, the class facilitators developed a brochure that explained the methods discussed. One of the lessons learned was that even in-house materials needed to be evaluated for appropriateness for all employees. "We created this little booklet in January but didn't review it for readability," recalls Kars. "We were pushing it out to everyone who participated in the class, and one of our leaders came back to us and said, 'My staff can't read this.' So we reviewed it, revised a lot of terminology, and now have a second version with easier-to-understand text." A term such as *outcomes* that is commonplace to management and quality improvement staff may not be understood by others in the organization; for Bronson's booklet, *outcomes* was changed to *results*.

Educators have also encountered resistance from both clinical and nonclinical staff who feel they are being asked to "dumb down" their language while speaking to patients. One problem is that many people equate education level with health literacy level and don't believe there can be comprehension issues with English-speaking patients who are high school or college graduates. Another problem is the comfort level that staff throughout a health care facility have with the terms they commonly use to communicate with each other. As Kars explains, "Those of us who work in a hospital have our own jargon, and we talk it all day, every day. So it's tough when you have to stop and think about what you're saying and break it down or use an analogy. If you're used to saying *myocardial infarction* all the time, why should you have to change to *heart attack*? Because it's more understandable for the patient."

The vignettes in the AMA Foundation video that show the experiences of actual patients have been helpful in promoting staff buy-in. Community members of the Patient and Family Advisory Council also help to bring home the communication needs of patients to management and staff. Some of them attend leadership meetings and tell stories of their care experiences. Others visit with residents in the pediatrics or internal medicine program each quarter and talk about what their needs are. "The residents understand that, even though they think they're doing their jobs because they're following protocols and doing what their attending physician requires them to do, they're really working with a patient who needs to be heard," says Kars.

Empowering Patients

Bronson has found various ways of promoting patients' well-informed participation in their care, including a systemwide campaign, a resource center that provides health information, and participation in a community literacy program.

It's OK to Ask

In 2006 Bronson began a campaign called It's OK to Ask. Based on The Joint Commission's Speak Up™ brochure, the campaign encourages patients to ask questions and be active participants in their care. Staff developed a brochure that included tips on how to communicate with caregivers, things patients should know about their medications, pain management and prevention of infections, and the importance of having an advocate. In 2008 this brochure was adapted to include the Ask Me 3 questions (*see* Figure 4-2, page 66). The revision was reviewed by the Patient and Family Advisory Council and then rolled out at Bronson Methodist Hospital. Now all inpatients and outpatients throughout the system receive a copy of this brochure.

At the same time that the It's OK to Ask and Ask Me 3 programs were being integrated into staff training and care delivery, staff began to explore ways to revise informational materials on warfarin and diabetes education materials for both outpatients and inpatients. The three questions from Ask Me 3 were incorporated into the revised materials, and the pharmacists who worked

Figure 4-2. Brochure from Bronson Healthcare Group's It's OK to Ask Campaign

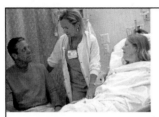

Patients and their families are the most important partners on the healthcare team. We expect you to ask questions, share information, and help make decisions about your care.

Three Key Questions
1. What is my main problem?
2. What do I need to do?
3. Why is it important for me to do this?

Reduce Infections
- Ask everyone that enters your room to wash their hands. Do not be afraid to remind your doctor or nurse. This helps to keep you safe from other people's germs.
- Ask family, friends and other visitors not to visit you when they are sick.
- Make sure to get your flu or pneumonia vaccine from your doctor or local flu shot clinic.

Bronson Methodist Hospital
601 John Street
Kalamazoo, MI 49007
(269) 341-7654

bronsonhealth.com

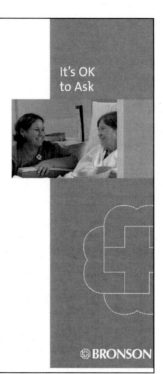

It's OK to Ask

Do You have an Advocate (Support Person)?
This family member or friend can help you keep track of everything going on.

This person can:
- ask questions for you
- take notes on what the doctor or nurse says
- stay with you while you rest
- help make sure you get the right medicine at the right time
- read over important documents for you
- make sure your wishes are honored, including life support
- update other family members and friends
- ensure you get proper care and instructions for when you leave the hospital

Important Documents
- Do you have a Durable Power of Attorney for healthcare?
- Do you have an Advanced Directive?

If not, please visit Important Documents on the Patient & Visitor Info section of bronsonhealth.com.

BRONSON

BRONSON

At Bronson, we want patients and families to be involved in their care. We want to partner with you and your family on choices that affect your hospital stay.

Please ask questions and speak up if you have concerns. If you do not understand, ask again. Talking with the doctor, nurse or other care provider helps make sure you and your family member get the best care possible.

You Are Part of the Team!
- Get to know us. These are the people who will be taking care of you or your loved one. Bronson staff should say their name when they enter the room. They also wear name badges. Ask what their job is. Many have special training you may want to know about.
- Talk about patient and family medical history. Share copies of medical records.
- Agree on exactly what will be done during each step of you or your family member's care. Make the decision with the doctor.
- Write down important facts. Keep track of any questions you may have.
- Ask the doctor how a new test or medication will help. More tests or medications may not always be best.
- Ask for test results and what they mean.
- Know what the plan is and how long you will be at Bronson. Talk about what to expect when you leave and how you should feel. Family members need to know what to do too.

Medication Safety
- Tell doctors and nurses about all of the medicines, over-the-counter drugs, herbal supplements and vitamins you are taking.
- Tell the doctor and nurse about how you react to different medicines. Make sure to tell them about any allergies.
- Ask your doctor about each drug he or she prescribes and what it is used for. Go over any possible side effects. Make sure it is OK to take that drug with your other drugs.
- Make sure the doctor writes the name of the drug clearly. You and the pharmacist should be able to read it.
- Ask the nurse to tell you what kind of medicine he or she is giving you and what it is for. Make sure it is for you. If you are not sure, ask the nurse to double check.
- Your nurse should open all your medicines in front of you. Anytime you receive medicine, shot or intravenous (IV) fluid, the nurse or other provider should ask for your name and birth date. This makes sure the right medication is given to the right patient.
- Write down the time of day you normally take your medicine. Call the nurse if you do not receive it on time.
- Ask for how long the IV should last. Tell the nurse if it is dripping too fast or too slow

Tell a staff member if something does not feel right. Do not assume anything. Try not to feel embarrassed — this is your safety!

Pain Management
- Tell your doctor or nurse as soon as you are uncomfortable or in pain. Do not wait until it is really bad.
- Most pain can be controlled and will be addressed promptly. It is OK to ask again if you feel your pain has not been addressed.

Stop a Fall
- Ask for help, even if you think you do not need it. You may be taking medicines that make you dizzy or light-headed.
- Keep your call button within reach. Use it when you need help.
- Ask for help getting up, such as to go to the bathroom.
- Make sure you have enough light to see. Keep your eyeglasses close.
- Tell your nurse about any wet floors or objects in your way so you have a clear, dry path.
- Wear socks or slippers with rubber soles. If you do not have any here, your nurse can get you a pair.
- Use your walker, cane, crutches or wheelchair when you are supposed to.

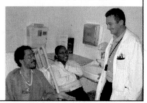

Source: Used with permission from Bronson Healthcare Group.

Bronson Healthcare Group staff adapted elements of the Ask Me 3 campaign and The Joint Commission's Speak Up campaign for the system's own campaign to encourage patient participation in care.

on the warfarin information developed a way to blend the information in their brochure (*see* Figure 4-3, page 68) with the verbal information they give to patients, using the Ask Me 3 questions as a foundation. "They'll walk in and talk about what's wrong, what we're going to do, and why you need to do it," describes Kars. "For example, 'There's a possibility of a stroke, so we're going to give you warfarin, and you need to take it consistently and continue to come back for your scheduled appointments because . . .'"

HealthAnswers

Providing health information that patients can understand is not confined to the educational materials given by clinical staff. Bronson HealthAnswers is an information center at Bronson Methodist Hospital. A part of the health sciences library, it is located in the medical offices pavilion in which 152 physicians have their practices. Anyone within the system can access the center by e-mail, through the Web site, or by phone; patients and members of the community can walk in at any time during service hours. Materials are available in English and Spanish, as well as at a variety of reading levels. The two full-time people who staff the center are not clinicians and only help users find general health information. They also help people use the two available computers and find reliable information that is appropriate to their needs. According to Kars, "A lot of people will say, 'I'm not comfortable using the computer,' and you don't know if that's true or if they can't read well and they don't want to tell you that. We use MedlinePlus® a lot because it gives people choices. It has a whole section of easy-reading materials and the tutorials about diseases, procedures, staying healthy, and tests, which are excellent pieces that anyone can use."

MedlinePlus is also a recommended component on the laptop computers that the hospital makes available to patients on the general medical, general surgery, pediatric, and antepartum units. Originally established with only a few laptops distributed by HealthAnswers staff on an as-requested basis so that patients could keep in touch with family and friends via e-mail, the program became so popular with both patients and staff that Bronson was prompted to keep five or six in the center and to place

four or more permanent laptops on each unit. Children can do homework, and patients and families can look for information on diseases, proposed treatments, and recommended tests. The HealthAnswers staff have created a "cheat sheet" for users so they can establish free e-mail accounts and research health facts. Kars sees the objective role that staff play in guiding patients toward reliable resources as invaluable: "Someone will say, 'I found this on the Web,' and the staff member then asks, 'Can you show me where you got it? Have you looked at who wrote the information? Here are some things to be aware of. If they're advertising a lot of things on that Web site, you may need to talk to somebody else about what other things are available. Always remember that your physician is the person who knows the most about your health.'" Bronson also offers classes on how to find good health information at the information center.

The HealthAnswers staff also provide price information for diagnostic testing, treatment, and procedures. Patients can use this information to better understand the costs of their health care and make informed choices.

Ready to Read

Since 1997 Bronson has been part of a community-wide emergent literacy program called Ready to Read, which is part of the national Reach Out and Read program. This proactive approach emphasizes the importance of reading to children as early as possible to promote brain growth and vocabulary development. As one of the cofounders of Ready to Read, Bronson gives books to newborns when they leave the hospital as a message to parents to encourage them to read to their babies. Every pediatric practice gives books to babies at wellness checkups, and practitioners tell parents about the importance of reading to their children. Books are also distributed at a guidance clinic and the local food bank, and there are volunteer readers at various community centers where children are likely to be. "We see low literacy as a generational problem," explains Kars. "If kids grow up in a family that doesn't read and doesn't have books in the home, they're not going to gain needed skills, and they're not going to do well in school. The emergent literacy program is something we started

Figure 4-3. Warfarin Brochure Revised for Easier Readability

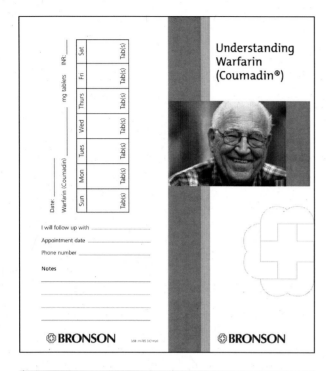

Understanding Warfarin (Coumadin®)

Date: _____

Warfarin (Coumadin) _____ mg tablets   INR: _____

	Sun	Mon	Tues	Wed	Thurs	Fri	Sat
	Tab(s)	Tab(s)	Tab(s)	Tab(s)	Tab(s)	Tab(s)	Tab(s)

I will follow up with ....

Appointment date ....

Phone number ....

Notes

....

....

....

⊕ BRONSON   b59 m785 3(1410)

⊕ BRONSON

Key Questions

1. Why am I taking warfarin (Coumadin®, Jantoven®)?
   – To keep from getting a blood clot

2. What do I need to do to take this medication safely?
   – Take my medicine at the same time each day
   – Watch for signs of bleeding
   – Make sure everyone knows I am taking the drug warfarin
   – Keep an up-to-date medication list
   – Keep my diet steady
   – Have my blood tested regularly

3. Why is it important to take warfarin safely?
   – To keep from getting a blood clot and reduce side effects

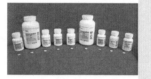

Watch the video "Warfarin and You" online at bronsonhealth.com

What is Warfarin?

Your doctor wants you to take the drug warfarin. Warfarin is the generic name for this drug. You may have also heard it called Coumadin® or Jantoven®.

Warfarin can help stop blood clots. It can also keep clots from getting larger. Sometimes blood clots form on surfaces of blood vessels due to damage to that blood vessel. Others form in the heart due to damage in the heart. When blood clots form, they can break off and move to other parts of your body such as your arms, legs, lungs and even your brain. If a blood clot blocks a blood vessel, it can stop the flow of blood, damage tissue, and can even cause death.

This brochure will tell you what to expect when you take the drug warfarin. If you have questions, ask your doctor, nurse or pharmacist.

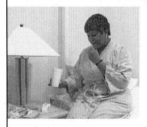

Taking Warfarin

Warfarin is a safe, yet powerful, drug. Please be careful how you take it.

- Do not take more than the dose prescribed by your doctor.
- Keep your pills at room temperature and away from heat, moisture and direct light.
- Take your dose at the same time each day. It is helpful to make this part of your daily routine.
- If you forget to take a dose, take it as soon as you remember, unless it has been more than 12 hours since your usual dose time.
- Do not take a double dose of warfarin the next day to make up for the missed dose.
- If you forget a dose, write it down. At your next visit, tell your doctor or pharmacist about the missed dose.
- If you are not sure whether you should take a dose, call your doctor or pharmacist.

Side Effects

Warfarin has been used for more than 50 years. It is a safe drug and is well tolerated by most people. However, some patients do have side effects.

Common Side Effects

These are side effects that you may experience. It is probably OK to keep taking your medicine. If you are not sure and something does not seem right, call your doctor or pharmacist.

- Gum bleeding while brushing teeth
- More nosebleeds than usual
- Easy bruising
- Bleeding after a minor cut that stops within a few minutes
- Menstrual bleeding that is a little heavier

Serious Side Effects

These side effects are very serious. If any of these happen, call your doctor or pharmacist right away.

- Red, dark, coffee or cola colored urine
- Bowel movements that are red or look like tar
- Bleeding from the gums or nose that does not stop quickly
- Vomit that is coffee-colored or bright red
- Anything red in color that you cough up
- Severe pain, such as a headache
- Sudden appearance of bruises for no reason
- Menstrual bleeding that is much heavier than normal
- A cut that will not stop bleeding within 10 minutes
- A serious fall or hit on the head
- Dizziness or weakness

Things to Remember

- Take your dose at the same time each day. If you miss a dose, take it as soon as you remember, unless it has been more than 12 hours since your usual dose time.

- Never double up doses if you miss a dose.

- Call your doctor or pharmacist if you notice any signs of bleeding or illness.

- Remember to tell all your doctors, including your dentists, that you are taking warfarin.

- Tell your doctor and pharmacist about all of your medicines, vitamins, herbal and dietary supplements.

- Try to keep your diet moderate and consistent. Eat the same amount of vitamin K each week.

- Go to your blood test appointments.

Resources:

Bronson Anticoagulation Clinic
601 John Street
Medical Office Pavilion, M–425
Kalamazoo, MI 49007
(269) 341-7909

Bronson Outpatient Pharmacy
601 John Street
Medical Office Pavilion, 1st Floor
Kalamazoo, MI 49007
(269) 341-6990

Bronson Pharmacy Mattawan
52375 N. Main Street
Mattawan, MI 49071
(269) 668-6205

Agency for Healthcare Research and Quality (AHRQ)
"Your Guide to Coumadin®, Warfarin, Therapy" www.ahrq.gov

Watch the video "Warfarin and You" online at bronsonhealth.com

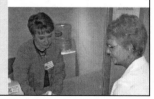

Source: Used with permission from Bronson Healthcare Group.

Bronson Healthcare Group's patient brochure on warfarin shows how the information has been presented to maximize usefulness and comprehension. The Ask Me 3 questions are answered briefly first and are then expanded on in the rest of the brochure. Space is given for patients to write down their dosing schedule, their physician's name and contact information, and notes from their discussion with the pharmacist who presents the information.

long before we started the health literacy program, but it fits into that."

Learning from Experience

As Bronson's various health literacy efforts have grown over the years, staff have learned important lessons through trial and error. Among the factors Kars lists for success are having executive and physician champions who make health literacy as a priority. "Our vice president for patient quality care and safety is our administrative champion," she comments. "She is the one who looked at the IOM aims and contacted people in the organization to ask them to head up a health literacy task force. Without her and the vice president for community affairs and development, this wouldn't be happening. They can push things out, address different segments of the population that I might not be able to reach. They also know the politics of the organization on a different level and can point things out. We also have a medical staff champion who's on the Continuum of Care Committee. He talks to the physicians, who see themselves as running the ship. He says, 'We have to work at this.'"

It is also important to build relationships with personnel from across the organization. Kars, who is a librarian without a clinical background, has built alliances with clinical staff and people in the education services department who understand the problems presented by poor health literacy. They are also familiar with The Joint Commission requirement that education and barriers to education (such as low health literacy) be documented in patients' charts. These people can push others toward awareness of literacy issues and the need for better communication.

Bronson also plans to find a way to measure how effective their various efforts are. The system currently uses a patient satisfaction survey that includes four questions pertaining to whether the information received from a physician or nurse was understandable and useful. Although scores have been fairly high, staff have not looked at the survey results over time to evaluate whether satisfaction improves as initiatives increase and more staff training is done. This would tell them whether staff are using the communication skills being taught.

"It's hard for health care organizations to keep momentum because there's so much going on all the time. We're constantly looking for better ways to do things, and there's not a lot of downtime," notes Kars. "But it all comes down to understanding your patients, knowing that if they don't understand the information, it's not their fault but yours. You have to form relationships and just keep at it."

CASE STUDY: EMORY UNIVERSITY

The earlier health care professionals of every discipline are introduced to the concept of health literacy, the more likely they are to integrate it into their normal patient care activities. However, based on the current literature, the number of schools that have set up curricula to address this need is still limited. In 2004 Emory University School of Medicine in Atlanta developed a program to educate medical residents about both health literacy and the appropriate communication skills for working with patients who have low health literacy.

The need for such education was identified in a preliminary study conducted by faculty in the school's Department of Internal Medicine. Medical trainees were given a written case study about a patient who was readmitted to the hospital for heart failure and asked to comment on what they thought were the underlying factors for the readmission. "They scarcely thought of health literacy as an issue, even when there were clear prompts that the patient may have had limited literacy skills," recalls Sunil Kripalani, M.D., M.Sc., then assistant professor of medicine at Emory and currently assistant professor and chief of hospital medicine at Vanderbilt University. "I was struck by the lack of attention that health care providers were paying to the issue of low health literacy. They didn't seem to be fully aware of it and didn't have the types of skills typically recommended for low-literacy communication. We decided to change that." Kripalani's study also found that only 25% of the medical residents included health literacy in their patient assessments, and just 4% of the patient care plans included elements that targeted literacy-related issues.

Doing the Preliminary Work

Three physicians and an educator who was experienced in both health literacy and physician education developed the training program at Emory. The actual creation of the program components took approximately three months, but other considerations also needed to be dealt with early in the process.

Audience Level and Integration of Curricula

"One of the initial decisions we faced was what the appropriate point of intervention would be—third-year medical students, fourth-year medical students, interns, residents," says Kripalani. "Intervening at the first or second year of medical school with this educational model would have been inappropriate. At Emory, first- and second-year medical students hadn't yet learned how to interview a patient, and to ask them to do more advanced communication skills would have been setting the cart before the horse. I wanted an audience that already knew how to interview patients and was ready to build on that knowledge. So that narrowed the pool to third-year medical students and up. Fourth-year students seemed to have enough of a comfort level with interviewing to learn about addressing health literacy."

Kripalani spoke with the director of the fourth-year clerkship in internal medicine to look at the possibility of integrating health literacy education at that point, but the time needed for the training didn't fit well with the existing curriculum: "One of the tensions in academics is there's so much material that you're supposed to teach and there's a limit on the amount of time that the trainees can be present." It was then decided to present the training to all internal medicine residents. This group had workshop time available that would allow health literacy training during their ambulatory care rotation, and the 8 to 12 housestaff per workshop were considered a good number for the educational model.

Getting Buy-In

The development team had little trouble convincing the faculty in charge of the curriculum that health literacy was an important addition to medical training. The three physicians involved were all from the Division of General Internal Medicine, and the internal medicine residency seemed an ideal place to focus on communication. As Kripalani explains, "In internal medicine, you'll typically spend 20 minutes with a patient. There are a lot of other disciplines where you may only spend 5

Figure 4-4. Components and Timing for Health Literacy Program

Day 1	Introduction	5 minutes
	Standardized patient encounters	25 minutes
	Health literacy workshop	90 minutes
Day 2	Video feedback session/behavioral prescription	20–25 minutes
	Program evaluation	5 minutes

minutes, and these encounters may be more focused on information gathering and physical examination rather than interpersonal communication and patient education."

However, an area where communication is particularly important to all physicians is the informed consent process. Particularly when invasive procedures are involved, being able to help the patient understand what will be done, why, the risks and benefits, and so on is crucial. "I've seen in my own practice that when surgeons talk about informed consent, they *really* talk about informed consent," notes Kripalani. "Informed consent is a perfect venue to showcase health literacy–related topics for procedural specialties."

Putting the Program Together

Evidence-based recommendations from experts in the health literacy field formed the foundation of Emory's educational model. Many of these recommendations—including teach-back and the use of visual aids and plain language—have been covered in detail in Chapter 3 of this book. The health literacy program consisted of an introduction and four main components (*see* Figure 4-4, above).

The program was implemented at Grady Memorial Hospital in Atlanta, Emory's primary teaching facility. Ninety-three first-, second-, and third-year residents participated in the program as part of their ambulatory care rotation curriculum from February to June 2004.

On the first day, the instructor gave a brief introduction to describe the topics to be covered in the health literacy workshop and to give out materials for residents

to review before they took part in the standardized patient encounters. After looking at the materials, the residents were divided into two groups.

Videotaped Encounters with Standardized Patients

As with most medical schools, Emory had a pool of actors who were accustomed to playing the role of patient, most often in the context of simulating specific physical illnesses. The development team e-mailed the pool and described what would be required of standardized patients for this program. Several people applied and participated in initial orientation and training sessions. One was deemed unsuitable because he was too aggressive and assertive. "We wanted people to be more subtle so the residents would have to pick up on cues that a typical patient would offer," explains Kripalani. "We also had some people with no prior acting experience. One of the best was someone who was just a friend of one of the actors. But all of them had experience as patients and had felt overwhelmed by information at some point in their own lives, so it was easy for them to get into the role." That role was of an adult with a high school education and limited health literacy. The patient participants were also trained in how to give residents feedback on their interviewing and communication skills.

The 10- to 12-minute patient encounters were held in examination rooms equipped with video cameras, notepads, pens, and patient education handouts. Seven rooms were used at a time. The first group of residents completed their scenarios while the second group took a break. The residents were asked to explain the diagnosis of a common condition (such as hypertension or hyperlipidemia) to the patient and counsel him or her on necessary lifestyle changes, medications, and possible side effects. After the first group's sessions were completed, those residents took a break and the second group came in.

Workshop

All residents participated in the 90-minute health literacy workshop, which was led by a faculty facilitator. The workshop comprised the following:

➤ An overview and definition of health literacy

➤ A discussion of how health literacy relates to patients' knowledge and behavior, health care costs, and patient outcomes

➤ A clip from the AMA Foundation's health literacy tool kit video

➤ An identification of indicators of low health literacy

➤ Communication techniques recommended for use with low-literacy patients

➤ Small-group breakout sessions to practice techniques

The development team took examples from many sources of evidence-based practices. "We looked at what other people were doing," says Kripalani. "For example, with the AMA program, we tried to hone it down to what would be the most important 30 minutes for medical trainees."

Communication skills focused on using plain language instead of medical jargon, eliciting questions from patients effectively, and using teach-back to confirm patients' understanding. All of the residents were encouraged to participate in discussions about any prior experiences with low-literacy patients and what communication problems they had encountered.

During the breakout sessions, residents were separated into groups of three to practice communication techniques through role play. They took turns playing the physician, the patient, and an observer (who provided feedback). The scenario in this case involved the physician explaining a diagnosis of mitral regurgitation.

Feedback from Faculty

Within three weeks of the first training day, residents were scheduled for a feedback session on their standardized patient encounter. This session took place with a faculty member whenever schedules permitted. "In many ways, this was the most memorable and valuable part of the program for the trainees—learning by doing and getting feedback on it," notes Kripalani.

The videos of the encounters were converted to CD-ROMs so they could be played back on computers and used as reference during the feedback sessions. The videos included both the patient encounter and a critique from the participating actor that was taped after the encounter. During the feedback session, the instructor offered both positive and constructive comments, taking the resident through the video and pointing out instances where language might have been simpler, behavioral cues that indicated how well the patient understood what was said, opportunities for using teach back, and so on. He or she also demonstrated methods to improve patient education exchanges.

When the instructor was finished, the resident was asked to write down two or three specific actions he or she planned to take in order to improve his or her communication skills. This "behavioral prescription" was written on the back of a small card that summarized the main points presented in the workshop on the other side. The card could easily fit in a pocket and be carried for reference.

Resident Evaluations

At the end of the feedback session, residents were asked to complete a program evaluation form consisting of 12 questions. Responses were uniformly positive, with 100% of respondents saying that the topic was relevant to their clinical practice and that the skills they'd learned were applicable to care delivery, 98.8% saying that the educational model was effective, and 96.3% saying that the program should be repeated.

Kripalani believes it is important to get feedback from learners: "The suggestions they had were operational, such as how much time to spend on one topic versus another. For example, we found that the second- and third-year residents really didn't want to do a lot of background on health literacy and how it impacts patient care. Once you told them, they said, 'Okay, I get that. Let's move on.' But the interns wanted a bit more of that."

Refining the Process

There is some question about whether it is better to teach health literacy as a stand-alone subject or to integrate it into the overall curriculum. As Kripalani comments, "When you teach trainees, you need to be aware that information decays over time, so you have to reinforce it. The ideal model—whether for medical, nursing, or pharmacy trainees—would probably be to introduce [students] to the concept of health literacy very early in their education. They're still talking like normal people, and they haven't yet gotten to the point where they think they have to communicate in technical jargon because that's what they see other people doing. Catch them early, make them aware of it; a lecture format would be fine for that." He recommends following up with the topic after students have acquired basic communication and interviewing skills. The type of program used at Emory, in which students can focus on the practical aspect of health literacy, would be preferable at that stage.

Reinforcement can take place in different ways. One would be to have a broad range of faculty members who are attentive to health literacy, so that it's one of the things they talk about, when appropriate, as they're precepting. The trainees then see that health literacy is not the pet project of one or two instructors; if all of the faculty keep talking about it, it must be a high priority.

Another way to reinforce learning is through problem-based learning, a prevailing educational model for medical students and residents. This model involves calling small groups of people together to discuss a case and talk about different aspects of it. Although these discussions tend to focus a lot on disease management and physiology, Kripalani points out that other elements, such as effective communication, may also be included: "Say there's a module on prostate cancer screening. You

can talk about digital rectal exams and PSA, but you might also have 10 minutes of the conversation be about how you would communicate clearly with the man about the options for prostate cancer screening. You keep coming back to the concept of health literacy and clear communication in these other venues to reinforce and extend the knowledge that people have already acquired."

Adapting the Program for Other Uses

Although the training program described here was originally designed for medical residents, the basic elements can be applied to different audiences such as nursing or pharmacy trainees or even established clinicians. To adapt the program effectively, educators would need to consider the intended audience members' level of comfort and experience with interviewing and counseling patients, their interest in health literacy, and their willingness to alter their existing communication techniques.

For example, the development team at Emory was asked to adapt and use this educational model for a research study funded by the Agency for Healthcare Research and Quality (AHRQ) and the Robert Wood Johnson Foundation, which involved training pharmacists in principles of clear health communication, equipping them with certain educational tools, and then testing the effectiveness of that training in a system-oriented study. Although the evaluation stage of this project is still forthcoming, the team found that there were distinct differences in working with this new audience. "The pharmacists represented a broader age base, whereas the medical residents were all young, had similar learning styles and levels of adaptability, and were there to learn," states Kripalani. "The practicing pharmacists varied quite a bit in how set they were in their communication patterns, how open they were to change, and their awareness of health literacy."

Adapting the program for a National Council on Quality Assurance webcast for primary care physicians required similar considerations. According to Kripalani, "Again, it was an audience of practicing physicians who weren't really in learning mode anymore. It was still successful though, because we tied health literacy into specific examples that they raised from their practice. We were able to engage them in topics that mattered to them individually, while still using some of the general principles and educational concepts we knew were important."

Notes

For more detailed information on the 2004 study of this training program, see "Development and Implementation of a Health Literacy Training Program for Medical Residents." *Medical Education Online*; http://www.med-ed-online.org/pdf/T0000097.pdf.

For information on the adaptation of the program for pharmacy staff, see Kripalani S., Jacobson K.L.: *Strategies to Improve Communication Between Pharmacy Staff and Patients: A Training Program for Pharmacy Staff.* AHRQ Publication No. 07(08)-0051-1-EF. Agency for Healthcare Research and Quality, Oct. 2007. http://www.ahrq.gov/qual/pharmlit/pharmtrain.htm.

CASE STUDY: GRADY HEALTH SYSTEM

A major factor in anyone's level of health literacy and access to care is understanding the language spoken by health care professionals and used in written materials. Making interpretation services available on a 24-hour basis and ensuring that staff use those services consistently can be problematic for many health care organizations. In-house staff versus contract agencies, face-to-face encounters versus telephone or webcam—these are only a few of the considerations that need to be addressed. Grady Health System, based in Atlanta, has established a Department of Multicultural Affairs (DOMA) that deals with all these questions.

Grady is a comprehensive system composed of Grady Memorial Hospital (a 953-bed teaching hospital), nine neighborhood health centers, a cancer center, an infectious disease program, a 354-bed rehabilitation center, a Level I trauma center, a burn center, and Georgia Poison Control. It serves a diverse population with varying levels of both functional and health literacy. Twelve percent of patients have limited English proficiency (LEP), and of this group, 90% are Spanish speaking. This makes health literacy and interpretation services high priorities for Grady.

Laying a Foundation

The DOMA primarily addresses cultural and linguistic barriers that can interfere with good patient outcomes. It has three main areas: (1) Language Interpretive Services, which addresses language access and includes both interpretation and translation services; (2) multicultural programs, which focus on community outreach and education; and (3) the International Medical Center. Health literacy is integrated into the various facets of the DOMA's work, as well as that of many other departments and groups within the system. For example, risk management personnel have worked with different departments, including the DOMA, to develop a consent form policy pertaining to health literacy. The policy states that consent forms must be written at a third-grade level, talks about teach-back, and requires that people who don't speak English or who are deaf have a qualified interpreter to help them read that consent form and verify their understanding.

Risk management, facilities management, and the DOMA also work together on signage at Grady Memorial. Instead of having signs in different languages, symbols that everyone can understand are used to navigate the hospital. Currently in the pilot phase, the signage beta test site is the emergency department, which has the most traffic.

Patient safety personnel have promoted the Speak Up campaign, emphasizing to staff throughout the system that patients need to be encouraged to ask questions if they don't understand or think staff members are doing something wrong. Grady holds a patient safety week in the atrium of Grady Memorial each year to educate patients about such topics as avoiding adverse events. "We talk to the LEP patients about the need for them to understand what they're being told and ask for a qualified interpreter," says Sandra Sanchez, M.S., director of Grady's DOMA. "With the English-speaking patients, we talk about health literacy. We tell them they have the right to ask questions when they don't understand."

Along with the departments that have made health literacy a priority, various physicians champion improvement as well. For example, there is Grady's chief of staff, who supports all initiatives pertaining to patient safety, communication, and literacy; the medical director of the International Medical Center; and the physician in charge of some of the neighborhood health centers. These and other proponents help raise awareness of health literacy needs among their peers and facilitate the integration of efforts, such as interpretation services, into daily activities.

Meeting Interpretation and Translation Needs

Atlanta hosted the Olympic Games in 1996, after which the population—particularly the Hispanic population—grew considerably. Grady Memorial's chaplaincy department began recruiting Spanish-speaking volunteers in churches or at the hospital to help patients with limited English skills. In 1999 the director of patient advocacy took on the task of creating a department.

Interpretation Services

In 1999, when the first coordinator and first interpreter were hired, there was one desk that served as their office. The interpreter, who was bilingual but had no formal medical interpretation training, had a pager and was on call around the clock. The two-person department tried to cover all areas of the hospital, but the need was overwhelming. Although a few more people were hired to help, organizationwide support was missing, primarily due to a lack of recognition of the true need. At that time, most physicians thought using family members or staff members as interpreters was acceptable, and the patient safety issue of poor outcomes and adverse events stemming from poor communication was not yet well known.

In 2002 things began to turn around. The coordinator and the director of patient advocacy decided to make the service more valuable and more visible. Everyone in the department was trained as a medical interpreter and obtained a certificate in that field. Their skills were assessed, and those who did not pass the requirements were given additional training and opportunities for reassessment. "The point was not to get rid of anyone, but to have all the interpreters at the same level," explains Sanchez. The department began developing policies, procedures, and forms to ensure that all interpretations were documented and that the process was as easy as possible. Staff also created flyers about their services—which were handed out to everyone in the hospital, including patients, nurses, and physicians—to publicize the hours of operation, available services, and so on.

Thanks to the hospital staff's new awareness of the department and the city's growing population, the demand for interpretation services increased significantly. "Our peak time was probably in 2003," recalls Sanchez. "The CEO at that time gave us a lot of support. We met with him, and he said, 'If you had a million dollars right now, what would you do?' He let our imaginations fly."

One of the obvious needs was more interpreters, and the department continued to grow to its present size of nine full-time and three part-time interpreters. The requirements for current staff are much more rigorous than those for the first interpreter in 1999 (who is still a member of the department). One of those requirements is to go through training in medical interpretation, during which they learn about the interpreter's code of ethics, standards and protocols, the role of the interpreter in patient encounters, medical terminology, and cultural issues for the populations they serve. Their skills are assessed by Grady personnel before they are hired and then again after six months.

Continuing education to keep skills up-to-date is an important part of the job. The department has biweekly one-hour classes for interpreters on medical terminology and note taking. There is also an annual training session (*see* Figure 4-5, page 77). "It's like a miniconference that covers different topics—where the field is, how the profession has changed," explains Sanchez. "For example, this year we're going to cover a medical topic, hold a session on memory-building skills and a session on note taking, then have a panel on advocacy issues as they relate to interpreting. Everybody's required to go."

Providing Needed Coverage. In 2004 the department came up with the idea of establishing a call center to be used for situations that did not require an interpreter to be present. Interpreters who are on duty sign in, and when they are not providing services in person, they staff the call center. Grady personnel can dial the appropriate extension from anywhere in the hospital and be connected to the main call center line, which gives a variety of options. If no one is available in the call center or a language other than Spanish is required, the call goes to Language Line. Videoconferencing is available for those who need sign language.

Figure 4-5. Agenda for Interpreter Training

✚ **Grady Health System**
5th Annual Continuous Medical Interpreter Training

Building skills:
The Medical Interpreter's Strength

November 11th and 14th
AGENDA

8:30am –9:00am	Registration and breakfast
9:00am -9:15am	Welcome and Introductions
9:15am – 10:30am	Memory Skills Building
10:30am -11:45am	Note taking workshop
11:45am -12:30pm	Lunch
12:30pm – 1:45pm	Panel
1:45pm – 2:00pm	Break
2:00pm - 3:15pm	Medical Topic: Orthopedics
3:15pm - 4:45pm	Vocabulary Building Exercises
4:45pm – 5:00pm	Wrap up, closing remarks and evaluation

Source: Used with permission from Grady Health System.

This agenda shows the variety of topics covered in Grady Health System's annual training session for all interpreters. The highlighted medical topic varies from year to year, but the emphasis is always on both dissemination of current information and practical exercises to build skills.

Interpreters are on call at Grady Memorial 24 hours a day. The health centers operate during normal business hours, and the call center is available to all of them. Four of the centers have in-house interpreters of their own to deal with the high volume of patients they serve. If patients who have appointments at either the hospital or the health centers require interpreters in languages other than Spanish, Grady contracts with agencies that provide these services and arranges for them in advance.

Making Processes Efficient. The department has developed several ways to streamline processes to decrease the wait time for interpreters and ensure that patients who need interpreters get them. For example, cell phone–radios are now used instead of pagers to communicate in-house. "When we just had pagers, an interpreter had to look for a phone whenever he or she was called, and they pointed out that it was not efficient," says Sanchez. "So we switched to cell phone–radios and developed codes. Everybody has their own number—cell phone 1, cell phone 2—and uses that same number every day. Now the dispatcher can use the radio and just say, 'Phone 3, ATA,' and the interpreter says, 'Five.' That means that in five minutes he or she will be available or call back. We have different codes to make the conversations short."

Nursing education has trained all nurses to assess the functional literacy levels of patients and identify any language barriers or disabilities (such as deafness) that might hamper communication. A current project is having stickers in a distinct color placed in the chart of any inpatient who requires interpretation services. "We are trying to get them put on at admission, but it's not happening all the time yet," notes Sanchez. "Currently when the interpreter is called for the first time, he or she puts the sticker on the chart. It says, 'Patient Needs Interpreter,' and the language needed is written underneath." Because of the high volume of patients, something different is being designed for this area. The first page of the registration software has a field in the demographic information for preferred language and need for an interpreter. Staff are being asked to highlight these fields on the printouts they make for the patient charts instead of using a sticker.

To ensure that a sufficient number of interpreters is available during each shift, staff collect data on wait times. Using a spreadsheet format, the dispatcher records the time each call is received, the name and title of the caller, the time the interpreter is contacted by radio, the interpreter's name and the time he or she responds, and the wait time. "The average right now is about 20 minutes," comments Sanchez. "If we have five calls at the same time and only two interpreters, we ask a few questions to assess urgency." The number of calls that need to be answered by Language Line can also indicate a need for more interpreters during certain times.

Training Staff to Use Interpreters. All new employees—including clinical staff, support staff, and contractors—receive orientation on how to use interpretation services. A half-hour presentation tells them why they need a professional interpreter and the process for

requesting one. Everyone also receives a small brochure with instructions for using the call center, tips for working with on-site interpreters, and how Grady interpreters have been qualified (*see* Figure 4-6, page 79).

Ongoing education about the proper use of interpreters is also given to existing staff. "We try to have staff meetings in two areas a month where we talk about not using family members as interpreters," explains Sanchez. "Sometimes even after all this training, you still hear someone say, 'But if the sister/child/mother/friend speaks this language, why can't I use him or her?' We say, 'Imagine that you're talking about a sexually transmitted disease or drug use or finances. You don't want to tell your neighbor or anyone else about that.' And many of our assessments ask about those things. So patients may initially say, 'Yes, he or she can interpret for me,' but when they get in the exam room and hear these questions, they may realize that they don't want to disclose that information in front of other people." Specific examples like this often help staff understand why they need a professional interpreter.

Sanchez also sees how physician attitudes are affected by the health literacy curricula adopted by the two medical schools affiliated with Grady: "A lot of the residents and medical students try to address [health literacy] issues. For example, they come in and say they want an interpreter, whereas more established physicians don't see that need. Although the interpreters are supposed to interpret everything each person says, they're obligated to ask the patient to summarize what he or she understood during the session, even when that's not asked by the physician or nurse. Then the interpreter interprets the patient's response. At the beginning, there was resistance to this from some clinicians, but now they're accepting it and actually doing it more often. A lot of physicians are moving toward doing more for health literacy—whether because of school curricula, because they've seen others doing it, or because they feel it's policy. It's a work in progress."

Translation Services

Whereas *interpretation* refers to oral communication, *translation* deals with the written word. All Grady

Figure 4-6. Staff Brochure Outlining Interpretation Services

⊞ Grady Health System **Dept. of Multicultural Affairs** Language Interpretive Services **Services provided (24/7):** • On-site Spanish interpreters • Sign language interpretation via video conference • Telephonic interpretation for more than 150 languages. **Office: 404-616-9626** **Pager: 404-871-1196** For TDD telephones (telecommunications devices for the deaf), please call 404-616-9626 option 5 <div align="right">Page 1</div>	When requesting a Grady interpreter in person, please have the following information available: • Language needed • Type of interpretation (medical, admission, discharge, etc.) • Your name, title, area, extension/pager • Patient's name If after placing your request, the interpreter <u>is no longer needed</u>, please notify us at 404-616-9626, option 5 immediately. <div align="right">Page 2</div>	**When calling Language Interpretive Services (404) 616-9626 at Grady Health System, you will hear the following options:** **Press 1** for languages other than Spanish (over the phone)* **Press 2** para escuchar mensaje en español **Press 3** for registration, billing, appointments, customer service in Spanish (over the phone)* **Press 4** to communicate health or medical information in Spanish (over the phone)* **Press 5** to request Spanish interpretation in person, to schedule a sign language interpreter or any other reason. *You may be asked for your access code (Extension of clinical manager or supervisor) **Please remember to remain on the line.** <div align="right">Page 3</div>
Tips for working with an on-site interpreter: • Brief interpreter before entering the room. • Position yourself to maintain eye contact with the patient. • Address the patient, not the interpreter. • Use the first person "I". • Everything you say will be interpreted. • Use short sentences. • Avoid technical jargon. • Allow interpreter and patient to finish without interrupting. • Check for understanding. • Tell the interpreter when the session is over. • Do not ask the interpreter to do anything but interpret (i.e. cannot sign as witnesses) <div align="right">Page 4</div>	**All Grady interpreters adhere to the Code of Ethics established by the National Council of Interpreting in Health Care.** All Grady interpreters have demonstrated: • Proficiency in English and one target language • Proficiency in medical terminology in both languages • Medical interpreting training and knowledge of interpreter roles, standards and protocols • Awareness of the role of culture in medical encounters • Interpreting skills that support the provider-patient relationship <div align="right">Page 5</div>	Grady patients have rights, including the right to free language interpretation services. Joint Commission also requires the use of qualified interpreters Grady Health System staff and providers **SHOULD NOT**: • Use family members (especially children) or friends to interpret. • Use bilingual staff as interpreters unless they have been qualified to do so by Grady Language Interpretive Services. • Ask patients to bring their own interpreter. Access to language interpretive services is federally mandated under Title VI of the Civil Rights Act of 1964 and the Americans With Disabilities Act. <div align="right">Page 6</div>

Source: Used with permission from Grady Health System.

This brochure, designed to fit into employee badge holders, is passed out every week in new-employee orientation.

publications—whether they are education materials or forms—that are used by patients are reviewed to ensure that they are written at a third-grade level. All of these forms are also translated into Spanish. A multidisciplinary committee must approve all patient forms, which are bilingual, with the English and Spanish versions appearing on opposite sides. This format ensures that whenever an English version of a form is revised, the translation is revised as well. It also makes it easier for staff who do not read Spanish to identify the correct form from the English version.

Having different departments review each form helps ensure both readability and accuracy. For example, nurse educators look at the forms for such things as reading level and formatting (bullets, white space, and so on). If a form concerns medication, the pharmacy will look at it for information that must be written in specific ways. DOMA staff are responsible for having each form translated and often have forms that are considered vital documents reviewed by Spanish-speaking patients. According to Sanchez, "We get feedback for the Spanish versions because there are so many countries that speak Spanish; one word can mean many different things in different countries. Patient review is another way for us to determine if we're using words that everybody understands. Even though the translations are done by professional translators and reviewed by different members of the team of language interpretative services, we want to make sure that the patients who are going to be using the forms can understand them."

Educational materials are also produced in both Spanish and English. One handout actually originated as an aid for Spanish-speaking patients in the community. The two-sided sheet provided a checklist of questions that patients should ask their physicians during an appointment, as well as tips for preparing for a physician visit (for instance, bringing a notebook and current medications along). The original handout used the questions from Ask Me 3, but staff found that those did not cover all of the points important to the Hispanic audience, so they revised the list based on user feedback. They distributed the sheets at health fairs and through other outreach programs. Based on its success in this venue, the sheet has been translated into English and is now being rolled out at Grady Memorial in both versions (*see* Figure 4-7, pages 81–82).

Looking Ahead

As the DOMA continues to try to improve its services, a couple of special projects are on the horizon. One involves an existing volunteer program. Students from two Atlanta schools that offer medical interpretation training can choose to participate in a type of internship program at Grady. "They don't do medical interpretation; they do customer service types of interpretation such as billing or making appointments or helping people navigate the facility," Sanchez explains. "The people who have gone through the program love it and stay with us as volunteers after they're out of school." The students, who receive course credit for their work, are evaluated by Grady staff on their performance, attendance, and so on. In some cases, a school requires that students do a certain amount of actual interpretation, and one of the professional interpreters monitors them during the patient encounters. Sanchez wants to expand this program to other schools and to develop a more structured curriculum for the volunteers.

Another future project is establishing a process whereby the DOMA can get feedback from clinical staff on interpretation services. One proposed method is to have the interpreters carry survey cards and envelopes addressed to the department for distribution to clinicians after patient encounters. "It would probably be something with five questions at most so we can find out how we're doing and how we can improve," says Sanchez. "We're trying to think of a way to measure our performance beyond just wait times. Health literacy is so important, and we're always trying to do something better."

Figure 4-7. Patient Tips for Communication

✚ **Grady Health System**®
Department of Multicultural Affairs

**RECOMMENDATIONS FOR CLEAR COMMUNICATION ABOUT YOUR HEALTH
WITH YOUR DOCTOR OR HEALTH CARE PROVIDER**

BEFORE YOUR APPOINTMENT:

☐ If you need an interpreter, ask the doctor's office to make arrangements for your appointment.

☐ Always bring a notebook to write important information.

☐ If you think you may have a problem remembering or understanding the information, write it down. If appropriate, ask a family member or a friend to accompany you for help during your visit.

☐ On your notebook, make a list of concerns about your health to discuss with your doctor or health care provider.

☐ On your notebook, make a list of your symptoms. If you know, write what produces those symptoms and since when you started feeling them.

☐ Bring the containers of all the medications that you are taking, including natural remedies.

☐ Ask the name of the doctor or health care professional who will take care of you and write it down to have as a reference.

☐ Be sure to discuss any drug or food allergies that you have (even if you are not asked).

☐ Repeat the information and instructions given to you by your health care professional, to ensure that you understood correctly.

☐ Ask your doctor to clarify all the instructions. Write down all relevant information. Do not leave until all of your questions have been answered.

☐ Find out whom to call if you have questions.

☐ If you have questions about your medications, ask your pharmacist to give you detailed information or instructions.

ASKING THESE QUESTIONS MAY HELP TO:

√ Take care of you health.
√ Understand your health situation and treatment.
√ Save money and time by avoiding additional appointments.

√ Be prepared for medical exams.
√ Take your medications correctly.
√ Maximize the time of the visit.

YOU DO NOT NEED TO FEEL IN A HURRY OR ASHAMED IF YOU DO NOT UNDERSTAND SOMETHING. DO NOT LEAVE IF YOU HAVE DOUBTS.

Recommendations for Clear Communication between patients and healthcare professionals
Grady Health System-Department of Multicultural Affairs
Adapted from Xlodar and Ask me 3.
04/07

(continued on page 82)

Source: Used with permission from Grady Health System.

This list, available in both English and Spanish, gives patients clear, easy-to-follow tips for talking to health care professionals in any setting. Originally based on Ask Me 3, it was expanded to address the concerns expressed by community members.

Figure 4-7. Patient Tips for Communication (continued)

✚ Grady Health System®
Department of Multicultural Affairs

CONSEJOS PARA UNA COMUNICACIÓN CLARA SOBRE SU SALUD CON SU MÉDICO O PROVEEDOR DE SALUD

ANTES DE IR A SU CITA MÉDICA:

☐ Si necesita un interprete, pida que en el consultorio medico se le hagan los arreglos necesarios.

☐ Siempre traiga una libreta para escribir información importante.

☐ Si cree que tiene problemas para recordar o entender la información, escríbala. Si lo considera pertinente lleve a un familiar o amigo para que le ayude durante su cita médica.

☐ En su libreta, haga una lista de las preocupaciones sobre su salud para decírselas a su médico o proveedor de salud.

☐ En su libreta, haga una lista de sus síntomas. Si lo sabe, escriba que produce esos síntomas y desde cuando empezó a sentirlos.

☐ Traiga todos los envases de medicina que está tomando, incluyendo los de remedios naturales.

☐ Pregunte el nombre del médico que lo va a atender y anótelo para tenerlo de referencia.

☐ Asegúrese de decir si tiene alergias a medicinas o alimentos (aunque no se lo pregunten).

☐ Repítale a su médico la información y las instrucciones que le dio, para verificar que usted entendió correctamente.

☐ Pídale a su médico que le clarifique todas las instrucciones y escriba toda la información importante. No deje el consultorio hasta que se hayan contestado todas sus preguntas.

☐ Averigüe a quién puede llamar si tiene preguntas.

☐ Pídale al farmacéutico que le explique detalladamente cuando tenga preguntas sobre sus medicinas.

HACER ESTAS PREGUNTAS LE PUEDE AYUDAR A:

√ Cuidar de su salud.
√ Entender su estado de salud y su tratamiento.

√ Ahorrar tiempo y dinero de consultas adicionales.

√ Prepararse para pruebas médicas.
√ Tomar sus medicinas de la manera correcta.

√ Aprovechar mejor el tiempo de la consulta.

NO NECESITA SENTIRSE APRESURADO O AVERGONZADO SI NO ENTIENDE ALGO. NO SE VAYA A SU CASA CON DUDAS

Recommendations for Clear Communication between patients and healthcare professionals
Grady Health System-Department of Multicultural Affairs
Adapted from Xlodar and Ask me 3.
04/07

CASE STUDY: IOWA HEALTH SYSTEM

Spreading awareness about health literacy and adapting processes and written materials to make information easier for patients to understand can be difficult in a single health care facility; when dealing with multiple settings across a large geographic area, it can be even more challenging. The Iowa Health System (IHS) is the state's largest integrated health care system, comprising 10 large hospitals, 14 rural hospitals, and more than 400 primary care physicians. In October 2003 IHS initiated its Health Literacy Collaborative among its affiliate hospitals to address multiple dimensions of health literacy—interpersonal and written communications, the care environment, awareness, education and training, and collaborative partnerships. The collaborative's goal was to create a shame-free, patient-centered care environment that promoted effective communication to help individuals read, understand, and act on health information.

The impetus behind this move was a review of data on literacy levels in general. National figures showed that half of U.S. adults read below high school level, and the 1993 National Adult Literacy Survey data for Iowa demonstrated that 38% of Iowans read at or below that level. The system pulled up city-specific data from those areas where they have affiliates, and the percentages ranged from 30% to 50%. According to Mary Ann Abrams, M.D., M.P.H., health management consultant in the IHS Department of Clinical Performance Improvement and leader of the collaborative, "A lot of providers say, 'These are not our patients,' but when this many adults read at that level, you know that many of them *are* our patients. We don't just take care of the other 50%."

One of the underlying principles of the IHS collaborative is its emphasis on the universal nature of low health literacy rather than a focus on specific demographic groups. "This is not just certain people; anyone at any time can have difficulty understanding or remembering, even a highly educated member of the health care team," states Abrams. "If you're sick or in pain, if you're on medication or you've been up all night, if you've just heard the word *cancer*, if you've been sitting in a waiting room for three hours and you need someone to pick up your children—there are a hundred reasons why you may not be able to understand or remember something. We try to apply good communication principles to everyone and then focus additional effort on those who may really struggle."

Getting the Ball Rolling

The first step the collaborative took was to hold a series of health literacy workshops for representatives from the affiliate hospitals. Beginning in 2003 and running through 2004, the workshops used components of the AMA's Train-the-Trainer module, the AMA Foundation's health literacy tool kit, and the Institute for Healthcare Improvement's Model for Improvement. Each hospital's leaders were asked to select interdisciplinary team members from their institutions to participate, and most of those chosen were nurses, patient educators, and staff educators. Although no physicians were present, the teams were encouraged to identify at least one or two clinicians who might be willing to serve as early adopters and champions of such methods as teach-back.

Although the workshops highlighted taking training on health literacy back to the individual hospitals, they also focused on the need for action. "Providing education is important and necessary, but it's not sufficient to make a difference," notes Abrams. "So although they took the information we gave them back [to their facilities] and did lots of training, we asked them to actually work on implementing interventions."

The greatest barrier to the dissemination and acceptance of health literacy information and training in individual organizations seemed to be a lack of awareness and understanding of the topic's importance. To overcome this, nearly all of the teams used the AMA

Foundation's video in their presentations. Along with explanations of the barriers and issues to good communication and the evidence of the impact on patient outcomes, the video features vignettes of people who have had trouble understanding diagnoses, instructions, and so on. "They look just like people in our practices and hospitals every day," explains Abrams. "Almost universally, once that video is shown, the teams get good buy-in and support from their audience."

Another way the teams improved buy-in was to include a patient or an adult learner in their efforts. Even if they did not have one on the team itself, they invited an adult learner to make a presentation and tell his or her own story. Having local people talk about their experiences put "faces to the data" and helped practitioners see the need for clearer communication.

Implementing Interventions

The Health Literacy Collaborative chose several types of interventions for rollout in the system's hospitals (and later to its outpatient clinics, home health services, and staff development programs). These interventions included teach-back, Ask Me 3™ and promotion of a shame-free environment, and revision of written materials. The system provides leadership for the collaborative and works to make sure projects take into account the Centers for Medicare & Medicaid Services' (CMS) quality indicators, as well as Joint Commission priorities. Individual organizations chose their target patient populations and how the interventions could best be adapted for those populations. For example, one hospital focused its efforts on improving discharge instructions for heart failure patients.

Teach-Back

As described in Chapter 3, teach-back is a method in which a provider (such as a physician, nurse, or pharmacist) explains health information to a patient and then asks the patient to repeat that information back in his or her own words. Clinicians are often concerned about this type of intervention because of the extra time they imagine it will take. The IHS teams have tried to overcome this mind-set during training by asking physicians to try it one time with one patient. One of the physicians

decided to try it with the last patient of the day in his office, so he did not need to worry about people backing up in the waiting room. This took a great deal of pressure off and allowed him to evaluate the effectiveness and ease of the method. It is also much less threatening to try something new with one patient than to suddenly be told that it needs to be done with all patients beginning on a certain date.

Abrams has worked with residents in the system's teaching hospitals and found that predictions of difficulty and patient resistance were unfounded. "They're pleasantly surprised that it doesn't take as long as they thought, it wasn't hard to do, and the patient appreciates it," she says. "They're also surprised that Mrs. Smith didn't understand what she was supposed to do, even though they thought she did because she's a nurse or a teacher. Once they have that recognition, they see why this is important."

One of the reasons that teach-back does not take as much time as anticipated is that as providers become more familiar with the process, they tend to explain things more clearly up-front. Because they know that they are responsible for a patient "getting the answers right," they start to use plain language, focus on the most important information, and emphasize actions the patient needs to take.

Ask Me 3

The teams also introduced Ask Me 3 (the tool that gives patients three important questions to ask their providers) to their organizations. As with teach-back, staff and clinicians were surprised that this tool could be implemented fairly easily and did not take a great deal of extra time. The program was implemented systemwide, and hospitals used many different activities to integrate it into operations. The following are examples of such activities:

➤ Displaying Ask Me 3 materials in both waiting rooms and patient rooms
➤ Including Ask Me 3 notepads in patient gift bags
➤ Writing articles for hospital newsletters
➤ Focusing on Ask Me 3 during Health Literacy Month activities

➤ Adding Ask Me 3 links to hospital Web sites

The system's largest facility in Des Moines adapted the Ask Me 3 poster, keeping the three basic questions and adding text to encourage patients to use them. The same information is printed as a flyer that is included in the hospital's admission packet (*see* Figure 4-8, page 86). Nurses take it out and explain it to patients when they're admitted, with the idea that the flyer will become the central place for patients to write questions and that when physicians or nurses go into patients' rooms, they will write things there as well. "The flyers are coupled with the posters and staff participation, because if you just put up a poster and none of the staff know about it or support it, it just becomes another poster," explains Abrams. "It's not just posters and handouts. It's our people saying, 'Make sure you get your questions answered.' It's a culture tool."

Organizational culture and the atmosphere staff create is an important factor in whether patients feel empowered to ask questions and participate in their own care. The IHS collaborative does not routinely test for health literacy level because it can make patients feel self-conscious and reluctant to admit that they cannot complete the questions. IHS affiliates have worked to raise staff sensitivity to these issues, and some facilities have incorporated questions about how patients like to learn new things and how happy they are with their reading level into the nursing assessment. The goal is to pass this information on to other members of the care team, and some nurses have made referrals to adult literacy programs based on the answers.

Staff are also encouraged to offer to help patients complete forms when they are given out. For example, a nurse or physician's receptionist may say, "These forms are complicated. A lot of people have trouble with them. If you need help, just let me know. We help people with them all the time." This approach can be much more successful than waiting for patients to ask for help, because many do not wish to say they don't understand. Abrams suggests learning from the way the hospitality industry approaches guest interactions: "When people come within ten feet of you, you look up and smile; when they're five feet closer, you say, 'How are you today? Can I help you?' We think about all those things that make a subtle difference in the whole tone of a patient's experience of the encounter."

Finding their way through a facility can also be problematic for patients and family members, so some IHS hospitals have started to work with the New Readers of Iowa to try to improve navigation. One affiliate has a New Reader on the health literacy team, and this person goes through the facility and provides feedback on signage on an ongoing basis. Staff use his comments to suggest changes. Several New Readers went to the Des Moines hospital to participate in walking interviews. Staff instructed them to go from the main entrance to the cafeteria and talk about what they were seeing, how they made their decisions, what they were looking for when they got to a hallway intersection, and so on.

Written Materials

Most IHS facilities continue to work on improving the usefulness and readability of their forms and brochures. "A lot of people believe that health literacy is just about the written materials, and although that's an important part of it, it's not all of it," says Abrams. "On the other hand, revising written materials seems easier than other interventions in some ways, because you have certain principles to follow and you can judge reading level. It's a tangible thing. We were able to provide a couple of training workshops on reader-friendly materials, which were very well received. Many of the teams got started in that area because it's something you can do early on and see the changes fairly quickly."

Teams go about their changes in various ways. They either choose something they want to work on, such as diabetes information, or have interested staff members bring in things that they think need improvement. After these projects took off, they started helping other staff understand what it takes to create reader-friendly print materials, and many staff members now ask for revisions or drafts of new documents to be further along before they are brought to the team for final review.

Figure 4-8. Ask Me 3 Handout

❶ **What is my main problem?**
❷ **What do I need to do?**
❸ **Why is it important for me to do this?**
Questions for my doctor, nurse, pharmacist or therapist:

█▌ **IOWA HEALTH**
DES MOINES
Methodist • Lutheran • Blank
Working together. Making a difference.

We Believe:
The more you know about your health, the better.

We Want You to Ask:
Your doctor, nurse, pharmacist or therapist questions about your health.
Ask us to tell you in plain language:

❶ **What is my main problem?**
❷ **What do I need to do?**
❸ **Why is it important for me to do this?**

If You Don't Understand:
Tell us you don't understand.

We Want You to Understand.

█▌ **IOWA HEALTH**
DES MOINES
Methodist • Lutheran • Blank
Working together. Making a difference.

For More Information on Clear Health Communication go to www.askme3.org.
CQ 138   Questions provided by the Partnership for Clear Health Communication.

❶ **What is my main problem?**
❷ **What do I need to do?**
❸ **Why is it important for me to do this?**
Questions for my doctor, nurse, pharmacist or therapist:

Source: Iowa Health Des Moines. Used with permission.

Staff at Iowa Health Des Moines adapted material from the original Ask Me 3 to create this patient handout, which is included in each admission folder. The statements on the right side of the handout also appear on a poster that is hung in patient rooms to encourage questions and participation.

The one form that the system has worked on as a whole is the consent for surgery and invasive procedures. Staff quickly identified that many different forms were used at the different organizations, but they were all written at the college level. Because informed consent is so important, everyone felt that this was an area that should be addressed. The director of risk management led the work to adjust the reading level of the form in partnership with the health literacy teams, adult learners (the New Readers of Iowa), and the law department. The consent form is now at the seventh- to eighth-grade level, incorporating principles of reader-friendly print materials. The document is one page, two-sided, with lots of white space and bullets, and it incorporates a teach-back section. It was pilot tested at one affiliate and has continued to be rolled out at other IHS affiliates.

External Partnerships

Working with outside entities has helped IHS further its reach in disseminating information about health literacy. For example, the Iowa Medical Society, Iowa Pharmacy Association, Pfizer, and the Iowa Department of Health are only a few of the external partners that helped promote Ask Me 3 through training, newsletters, conferences, and public health efforts.

The system is also doing some work with Reach Out and Read, a program targeted toward children six months to five years old to promote early literacy skills to support school readiness and health literacy. IHS considers its participation with this group to be a strategy for primary prevention of low literacy and low health literacy among children. Besides being an early literacy promotion tool for children, it is a tool to open conversations with parents or caregivers, explore their reading comfort, and ask whether they like to read or would like to learn more about programs to help them read better.

Measuring Success

To collect baseline data and measure improvement after interventions were instituted, IHS used five questions from the Press-Gainey patient satisfaction survey pertaining to whether patients received explanations of tests and treatments, instructions about medications and self-care, and whether nurses and physicians kept them informed. Baseline data were collected from October 2003 to June 2004, and follow-up data were collected from July 2004 to May 2006. Patient satisfaction went up in all five areas, with the highest rate of improvement in the areas of test/treatment explanations and medication instructions.

IHS is currently shifting to the use of the Consumer Assessment of Healthcare Providers and Systems Hospital Survey as their measurement tool. This survey has been validated and is being used by most hospitals as part of the CMS quality initiative. The items in the survey have been publicly reported since April 2008, and some of them are used in the reimbursement formula for pay for performance. Out of the seven domains in the survey, IHS found four to be closely related to health literacy; these deal with (1) communication with nurses, (2) communication with physicians, (3) communication about medication, and (4) communication about discharge information. "We have always focused on top-box scores, because that's what you really want to achieve and that's what drives improvement and helps set you apart," notes Abrams. "CMS did a couple of years' worth of roll-in data, and that's going to be our official baseline. Then we asked each affiliate to shoot for a 5% improvement on their original score, and we did the same for the system as a whole. That's our new goal. The data were just released last spring, so we've been working on getting all that into an easy-to-read format.

"CMS is going to release rolling data, but because of the way they do it, it's going to be old—something released today would be from last year. We've been working with our IT people and vendors to generate our own data and look at it on a monthly basis for each affiliate so we can try to be more proactive. Although it will be a couple of months behind, it won't be so much that we can't see the results of specific interventions."

Moving Forward

Although the Health Literacy Collaborative technically ended after the first three workshop sessions, the teams chose to continue to meet. Additional workshops were held in 2005 and 2006, and rural hospitals and home health services were added to the mix. Today team members hold monthly conference calls to share information, concerns, issues, and success stories.

The collaborative emphasizes the importance of juggling the many components of health literacy. "I often call it a bundle," says Abrams. "You have to have several things in place, not just one. From our work in public health issues like smoking and obesity, we know that we have to bring several different forces or aspects of intervention together to help make an impact. You have to have providers on board; you have to make patients aware that they should ask questions; you have to have an environment that invites and supports questions; you have to have materials that are easy to read and provide good information; and you have to have systems in place that support all that. It's not a single intervention; it's more of a portfolio."

Keeping momentum high for any collaborative can be difficult over time and across geographic locations. IHS has added health literacy components to job descriptions, employee orientations, and competency assessments to highlight that it is a top priority throughout the system. In addition to reviewing patient satisfaction data, many team members feel that it is essential to keep patients and adult learners in the middle of related activities. Seeing the people who are directly affected by improvements in communication methods helps keep all caregivers interested in continuing those improvements.

One of the most important points is involving everyone in each organization and getting them to recognize that health literacy applies to all aspects of care. "It doesn't matter whether you're getting a chest x-ray as an outpatient or in the hospital, having a prenatal visit, or are elderly with lots of chronic conditions," states Abrams. "There's a recognition that there's a link between health literacy; high-quality, patient-centered, safe care; and decreasing health disparities. All those things are going to be increasingly important as drivers to improve health literacy both internally and externally."

CASE STUDY: MINNESOTA ALLIANCE FOR PATIENT SAFETY

Bringing about widespread improvement in health literacy requires the collaboration of health care organizations, clinicians, public health and community programs, adult education and literacy experts, and many others. The Minnesota Alliance for Patient Safety (MAPS), a statewide safety coalition, was founded in 2000 by the Minnesota Hospital Association (MHA), the Minnesota Medical Association (MMA), and the Minnesota Department of Health to facilitate the development and dissemination of best practices pertaining to patient safety, including health literacy and medication tracking. Believing that adverse events are systems issues that occur in an interactive environment and therefore are not isolated, MAPS promoted a statewide model of a just culture that supports learning from mistakes yet holds individuals accountable for behavioral choices. In 2000 the coalition released its "Redefining the Culture for Patient Safety" brochure to explain key issues and terminology in patient safety.

Health literacy efforts surfaced early on. "We kicked off a 'patients as partners' campaign in 2002 and identified two tracks," recalls Tania Daniels, vice president, Patient Safety, MAPS. "One was a focus on patient engagement and education, and the other was provider education specific to health literacy." Although the approach to partnering with patients was broad, health literacy was an important component of the campaign. The group developed the "Patient Safety: Your Role" brochure in 2003. That same year, MAPS held provider training in general health literacy issues; in 2004 there was a train-the-trainer program based on the AMA Foundation's health literacy program. Six interdisciplinary teams from across the state attended the in-depth, two-day training sessions. Each team agreed to take on a specific health literacy–related project after going through this training. One of the teams was from HealthEast Care System, an integrated health delivery organization in St. Paul. Their chosen project was to reduce the reading level of the system's informed consent form from 12th grade to 5th or 6th grade, which later became a statewide project for MAPS.

Beginning the Change

Revising the form a health care organization uses for informed consent affects not only the form itself, but the process that goes with it, and this in turn affects those who conduct the process. Robert Moravec, M.D., medical director of HealthEast, became a champion of health literacy when he began reading about the evidence of low health literacy and its effects. "It wasn't in my job description or something I was asked to do," he says now of his initial involvement. "But in our downtown St. Paul hospital we have a fairly large Hmong population, and our Somali and Russian populations are increasing. Once I became aware of the need, I knew we had to start somewhere. The challenge is that this isn't really anybody's 'job.' It usually falls on the patient and family education coordinator, and with so much work to do, health literacy is easy to put off."

In 2004 HealthEast began work on its own informed consent process with a more literate consent form. Moravec partnered with a nurse from the Patient and Family Education Department, who had experience in surgery and in developing care brochures for patients, to simplify the 12th- to 14th-grade reading level. "It took a year to whittle down the language to the 7th- and finally the 6th-grade level," recalls Moravec. "Our biggest challenge was probably the surgeons. They thought it was too 'dumbed down' and that patients would feel they were being condescended to; it certainly didn't represent the surgeons and the language they would use. It took constant reminding that 'This isn't for you. You know what you're going to do. It's the patients who aren't sure what's going on, and you have to tell them.' By the time we actually got it through committee, it was a full year from the time we started working on it in our system. From there, it became a part of our practice."

Widening the Circle

Moravec wrote a resolution to the MMA House of Delegates in late 2005 that called on MAPS, the MMA, and the MHA to work on a statewide health consent form template. The resolution presented evidence about low health literacy, such as average adult reading level, and made medical leaders across the state aware of the problem. The issue was debated by MMA delegates, testimony was heard in reference committees, and the resolution was passed.

In 2006 MAPS commissioned an informed consent work group to create a standardized consent form for the entire state. The group comprised key stakeholders, including state health systems, hospitals, ambulatory surgery centers, clinics, the MMA, the MHA, the Minnesota Health Literacy Partnership (MHLP), health plans, insurers, the department of public health, and the community. Representatives ranged from physicians and nurses to patient advocates to educators to attorneys. Using consent forms and policies from HealthEast and Allina Hospitals and Clinics in the Twin Cities as a starting point, the work group met several times over the course of six months to identify what information needed to be covered in the form and decide on the easiest way to express that information. Group members were encouraged to get input from others and give feedback on the form throughout the process. Christine Norton, a retired English teacher and cofounder of the Minnesota Breast Cancer Coalition, served as a patient advocate for the group. "We would work on wording, content, and format at the meetings, then changes would be collated and sent to us for review and to gather feedback within our organizations," she remembers. "If I would attend a training session or meeting for the National Breast Cancer Coalition, I'd take the draft and show it to nurses and others who worked with patients and get their feedback. At the next meeting, committee members would be told how [the form] had been received."

At the same time that they were developing a consent form template, group members were also

working on a model policy to go with it. "Informed consent is an ongoing, interactive process," notes Moravec. "As the policy says, it focuses on more than just the signature. The process may begin in an outpatient office, include several providers, and occur over time rather than as a one-time information session prior to a procedure. It's expected that all treatment decisions are made only after a fully informed and shared decision-making discussion between the patient and the physician. The form should be the last step in the process."

After changes were made in April 2007 to coincide with requirements from the CMS, the model consent form and policy were given to the field for pilot testing. "It went out to hospitals, clinics, and surgical centers, so we had good representation," says Daniels. "And we received feedback from both providers and patients, which we incorporated in the final model." As with HealthEast's experience, there was again some resistance to the proposed templates. According to Becky Schierman, MMA manager of Quality Improvement, "Some physicians said, 'We have a lot of complex information we need to give patients, and this dumbs it down too much,' or 'My patients are smarter than that.' The MAPS form allows physicians to have an informed and relaxed conversation with patients in the clinic, rather than a rushed and ineffective conversation at the time of the surgery. When patients are in that stressful position, the majority of it's not going to be caught anyway."

Some facilities brought up time as a consideration for the new form. "At one meeting after the pilot test, someone said, 'We tried it, and the nurses who were using it said it was good but it takes longer than the old form,'" recalls Norton. "Two of us said simultaneously, 'That's because the patients are actually reading it now.'"

When the final changes had been made, copies of the informed consent policy and form (see Figure 4-9, pages 91–92, and Figure 4-10, pages 94–101) were distributed to every hospital and patient safety leader in the state. They were also posted on the MAPS Web site (http://www.mnpatientsafety.org), so that out-of-state facilities could use them as well. According to Moravec, "Each organization should look at it and ask, 'Does our

Figure 4-9. MAPS Template for Informed Consent Form

Minnesota Informed Consent

Consent form for surgery or invasive procedure

1. I, [print patient's name]: _____
    a. Agree that I will have [include both the medical term and patient words]: _____
    _____
    b. At [name of facility]: _____
    c. The reason for this procedure is [medical condition]: _____
    d. This will be done or supervised by: _____
    e. My doctor may have help from others. Help could include opening and closing the wound. Help might also include taking grafts, cutting out tissue, implanting devices. I have been told who will help, if known. The key team members that will assist are:
    Name/title: _____ Critical task: _____
    Name/title: _____ Critical task: _____
    Name/title: _____ Critical task: _____

2. I have talked to my doctor or health care team about:
    a. What the procedure is and what will happen.
    b. How it may help me (the benefits).
    c. How it might harm me (the most likely and most serious risks).
    d. The long-term effects the procedure might have.
    e. My other choices for treatment. The risks and benefits of those choices.
    f. What will likely happen if I say "no" to this procedure.
    g. How I might feel right after and how quickly I can expect to recover.
    h. What medicines will be used to manage pain or sedate me.

3. I agree that: (If I do not agree with a statement, I have crossed it out and initialed next to it.)
    a. I will ask questions.
    b. No one has promised me definite results.
    c. If it is best for me, my doctor may change the plan if they find other serious problems during the procedure.
    d. If I have "do not resuscitate" (DNR) wishes they will be put on hold during the procedure.
    e. Students and others may watch the procedure. This must be approved by this facility.
    f. Pictures or video may be taken. They may be used for medical or educational reasons only.
    g. Tissues or items removed from my body may be tested. They will be disposed of with respect. Unless I agree, tissues will not be used for research or sold.

MAPS Minnesota Informed Consent - form for surgery or invasive procedure   Page 1 of 2

(continued on page 92)

Source: Used with permission of the Minnesota Alliance for Patient Safety.

This two-page template presents a consent form for surgery and invasive procedures that can be adapted by hospitals, clinics, and ambulatory surgery centers. It is written at the fourth- to fifth-grade level, is formatted to promote ease of reading, and complies with the Centers for Medicare & Medicaid Services' Conditions of Participation.

Figure 4-9. MAPS Template for Informed Consent Form (continued)

h. If a staff person is exposed to my blood or body fluids, my blood will be drawn and tested for HIV and hepatitis. The test results will go:

- To me;
- In my medical record;
- To the exposed worker. This is to decide if treatment for the worker is needed;
- To the Employee Health Services Department and/or Infection Control at this facility; and
- To Minnesota health officials.

4. Blood transfusions:

I have been told how likely it is that I will need a blood transfusion. I know the risks and benefits of receiving blood products. My doctor and I talked about other options.

- You may give me blood (blood products) if I need them during my stay and if it is related to this procedure.
  - ◯ Yes
  - ◯ No

5. I understand that:

- **a.** I can change my mind. If I do, I must tell my doctor or team as soon as possible.
- **b.** The team members may change during the procedure.
- **c.** The team will double-check who I am. They will ask what I am having done. This is to protect me.

My questions have been answered. I agree to the procedure. My instructions and special needs are:

_____

_____

_____

Patient (or representative) signature/Relationship to patient	Date	Time

I have discussed the procedure and the information stated above with the patient (or patient's representative) and answered their questions. The patient or their representative consented to the procedure.

Physician or Provider signature(s)	Date	Time

Interpreter Name (if used)	Language/Organization	Time

I have verified that the signature is that of the patient or patient's representative. This form has been signed before the procedure.

Witness	Date	Time

MAPS Minnesota Informed Consent - form for surgery or invasive procedure

Page 2 of 2

Figure 4-10. Minnesota Alliance for Patient Safety (MAPS) Template for Informed Consent Policy

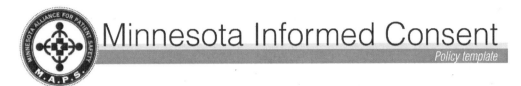

INTRODUCTION

In early 2007, the Minnesota Alliance for Patient Safety (MAPS) convened a work group to develop a statewide informed consent process. The impetus occurred when the Centers for Medicare and Medicaid Services (CMS) issued new Conditions of Participation (May 2004) and interpretive guidelines (April 2007). These guidelines required that a written informed consent process and form inform the patient of his or her health status, allow patients to be part of care planning, and provide the opportunity for patients to object to particular treatments.[1]

The right to make informed decisions is dependent upon the patient's and/or their representative's ability to fully comprehend the treatment to which they are consenting. The patient and/or their representative should receive information in a manner and language that is understandable to them. It was evident upon review of existing informed consent forms that the role of health literacy has not been considered and forms are often not comprehensible to the patient. During times of illness and stressful events, all patients could benefit from easy-to-understand health-care forms. A lower literacy level form does not preclude an in-depth conversation with those patients with higher levels of understanding. The form is designed to be at a minimum standard that all patients can understand. The MAPS template informed consent reads at a 4.5 grade reading level.

MAPS set out to develop a template form that every outpatient setting could utilize to facilitate the informed consent process and that every hospital and surgical center in Minnesota would accept as comprehensive informed consent documentation. The form includes all elements that make up a "well-designed informed consent form" as defined by CMS. This form also incorporates standards set by the Joint Commission and the Occupational Safety and Health Administration (OSHA).

MAPS envisions this form as Minnesota's universal documentation of informed consent and that health-care organizations statewide will use the informed consent form and accompanying policy with no variation. If this form is used, the MAPS logo should be included along with an organizational logo. However, at minimum, all of the elements must be included if represented as a MAPS form.

What is WRITTEN Informed Consent?

"Written informed consent" means that the patient and clinician have signed a document acknowledging that:

A. The patient has been provided information necessary to make an informed decision about a proposed medical treatment or procedure (the necessary information is listed on page 2 and 3 of this policy);

B. The clinician has discussed the procedure with the patient and answered the patient's questions; and

C. The patient consents to the procedure.

Purpose of the Informed Consent Process

Informed consent involves much more than just obtaining a signature. The informed consent process is ongoing and interactive. The process might begin in the outpatient office, involve several providers, and occur over time rather than occur as a one-time information session prior to procedure. It is expected that all treatment decisions will be made only after a fully informed and shared decision-making discussion between the patient and clinician.

---

[1] Requirements related to informed consent for hospitals are found in the Patients' Rights Condition of Participation (CoP) at 42 CFR 482.13(b)(2); the Medical Records CoP at 482.24(c)(2)(v); and the Surgical Services CoP at 482.51(b)(2). Interpretive guidelines for Tags A-0049 (Patients' Rights), A-0238 (Medical Records), and A-0392 (Surgical Services) replace the guidelines issued in May 2004.

(continued on page 94)

Source: Used with permission of the Minnesota Alliance for Patient Safety.

This nine-page template outlines a recommended process for communicating with patients who are to undergo surgery or invasive procedures. This process includes the physician's provision of information about the procedure and potential short- and long-term risks and benefits, followed by the patient's signing the appropriate form.

Figure 4-10. Minnesota Alliance for Patient Safety (MAPS) Template for Informed Consent Policy (continued)

The right to make informed decisions regarding care presumes that the patient has been provided information about his/her health status, diagnosis, and prognosis. Furthermore, it includes the patient's participation in the development of the plan of care, including consent to or refusal of medical or surgical interventions and in planning for care after discharge from the facility. Again, the patient or the patient's representative should receive adequate information, provided in a manner that they can understand. This assures that the patient can effectively exercise the right to make informed decisions.

INFORMATION THAT MUST BE PROVIDED TO THE PATIENT DURING THE INFORMED CONSENT CONVERSATION

For informed consent to be complete, the clinician must discuss in language and in a form that the patient can understand and must include at least the following information. The clinician must take reasonable steps to ensure that the patient understands the information provided (e.g., avoid technical jargon, ask whether they understand, encourage questions, use the "teach-back," method). For example, with "teach-back" method, the provider would ask the patient to restate what he or she understands to be the nature and risks of the procedure to be.

It is the facility's responsibility to assure, via established processes, that each patient or patient's representative is given information on the patient's health status, diagnosis, and prognosis.

The clinician's signature on the informed consent form or note in the record certifies the following information was provided.

A. The indications for the proposed surgery or other invasive procedure;

B. A description of the proposed surgery or other invasive procedure, including the anesthesia to be used;

C. Material risks and benefits for the patient related to the surgery or other invasive procedure and anesthesia, including the likelihood of each, based on the available clinical evidence, as informed by the responsible practitioner's clinical judgment. Material risks could include risks with a high degree of likelihood but a low degree of severity, as well as those with a very low degree of likelihood but high degree of severity. A relatively minor risk may be significant to a particular patient. If the clinician knows that the risk would be important to that patient's decision-making the clinician should discuss the risk with the patient;

D. Treatment alternatives, including the attendant material risks and benefits;

E. The probable consequences of declining recommended or alternative therapies;

F. Who will conduct the surgical intervention and administer the anesthesia, if known;

G. Whether physicians other than the operating practitioner, including but not limited to residents (see note below), will be performing important tasks related to the surgery or other invasive procedure, in accordance with the hospital's policies. Important surgical tasks include: opening and closing, dissecting tissue, removing tissue, harvesting grafts, transplanting tissue, administering anesthesia, implanting devices and placing invasive lines;

Note: For surgeries or other invasive procedures in which residents will perform important parts of the surgery or other invasive procedure, discussion is encouraged to include the following:

A. It is anticipated that physicians who are in approved post graduate residency training programs will perform portions of the surgery or other invasive procedure, based on availability and level of competence;

B. It will be decided at the time of the surgery or other invasive procedure which residents will participate and their manner or participation, and that this will depend on the availability of residents with the necessary competence; the knowledge the operating practitioner/teaching surgeon has of the resident's skill set; and the patient's condition;

C. Residents performing surgical tasks will be under the supervision of the operating practitioner/teaching surgeon;

(continued on page 95)

Figure 4-10. Minnesota Alliance for Patient Safety (MAPS) Template for Informed Consent Policy (continued)

    D.   Whether, based on the resident's level of competence, the operating practitioner/teaching surgeon will not be physically present in the same operating room for some or all of the surgical tasks performed by residents;

    E.   Whether, as permitted by state law, qualified medical practitioners who are not physicians will perform important parts of the surgery or administer the anesthesia, and if so, the types of tasks each type of practitioner will carry out; and that such practitioners will be performing only tasks within their scope of practice for which they have been granted privileges by the hospital.

PURPOSE OF INFORMED CONSENT FORM

Minnesota health-care facilities recognize a patient's right to give knowing, voluntary consent before receiving medical treatment. The purpose of the informed consent form is to verify that the process of informed consent has occurred between the patient and the clinician.

Signing the form should be the last step in this process. The informed consent form serves as a mechanism to confirm the patient understands the procedure and provides an opportunity for patients to ask additional questions about their procedure and the facility.

A properly executed informed consent form must be placed in the patient's medical record prior to surgery, except in the case of emergency surgery.

INFORMATION THAT MUST BE INCLUDED ON THE INFORMED CONSENT FORM

A "properly executed" informed consent form should reflect the patient consent process. Except as specified for emergencies in the hospital's informed consent policies, all inpatient and outpatient medical records must contain a properly executed informed consent form prior to conducting any procedure or other type of treatment that requires informed consent.

An informed consent form, in order to be properly executed, must be consistent with hospital policies as well as applicable state and federal law or regulation.

A "properly executed" informed consent form contains the following minimum elements:
    A.   Name of the hospital where the procedure or other medical treatment is to take place;
    B.   Name of the specific procedure, or other type of medical treatment for which consent is being given;
    C.   Name of the responsible practitioner who is performing the procedure or administering the medical treatment;
    D.   Statement that the procedure or treatment, including the anticipated benefits, material risks, and alternative therapies, was explained to the patient or the patient's legal representative;
    E.   Signature of the patient or the patient's legal representative;
    F.   Date and time the informed consent form is signed by the patient or the patient's legal representative.

A "well-designed informed consent form" might also include the following additional information:
    A.   Statement, if applicable, that physicians other than the operating practitioner, including but not limited to residents, will be performing important tasks related to the surgery, in accordance with the hospital's policies and, in the case of residents, based on their skill set and under the supervision of the responsible practitioner;
    B.   Statement, if applicable, that qualified medical practitioners who are not physicians who will perform important parts of the surgery or administration of anesthesia will be performing only tasks that are within their scope of practice, as determined under state law and regulation, and for which they have been granted privileges by the hospital;

(continued on page 96)

Figure 4-10. Minnesota Alliance for Patient Safety (MAPS) Template for Informed Consent Policy (continued)

C. Listing of the material risks of the procedure or treatment that were discussed with the patient or the patient's representative;

D. Name of the practitioner who conducted the informed consent discussion with the patient or the patient's representative;

E. Date, time, and signature of the person witnessing the patient or the patient's legal representative signing the consent form.

Documentation of Consent

When written consent is required, the clinician and patient must certify that the informed consent discussion has occurred and the patient is consenting to the procedure by signing the informed consent form. The form must include the minimum elements detailed on page 3, whether the facility from where the procedure is occurring or from the outpatient setting. The signed form must be placed in the patient's medical record.

1. Clinician's Signature: As a rule, the clinician must sign the informed consent form before the facility will permit the procedure to be performed. If the procedure is ordered by the clinician but is administered by a non-clinician (e.g., a blood transfusion or insertion of a central line) and the clinician cannot be physically present to sign the form prior to the procedure, the clinician may certify that the informed consent conversation took place and that the patient consented. The clinician must follow the facility's procedure for accepting an order by telephone.

   A. Verification of patient's signature by witness: When written consent is required, the facility should verify that the signature on the informed consent form is that of the patient. However, it is not necessary for a facility employee to witness personally the informed consent conversation between the clinician and patient nor the patient signing the form.

   B. Employee witness observes patient signing: A facility employee who observes the patient signing the form may verify that fact by signing the informed consent form as a witness to the signature.

   C. When signed out of employee witness's presence: If the form was signed by the patient out of the presence of a facility employee, an employee must confirm with the patient that the signature on the form is that of the patient and that the patient consents to the procedure. The employee must sign the informed consent form as a witness.

   D. When signed out of employee witness's presence and witness has signed: If another witness (e.g., a nurse in the clinician's office) has already signed the form, the facility employee may co-sign the form or note in the record that the employee verified the patient's signature.

When written consent is not required, the clinician may document the discussion and the patient's consent in a progress note stating that the informed consent process has occurred. Such a note certifies that the clinician has provided the information required and that the patient consented to the procedure. The clinician may – but is not required to – use the informed consent form to guide the informed consent discussion and to document the patient's consent, even when written consent is not required.

Physician's Responsibility

Obtaining informed consent is the clinician's responsibility and cannot be delegated to anyone else. A physician has the legal and ethical obligation to administer a medical treatment or procedure to a patient only if the patient has given the clinician informed consent to the treatment or procedure.

The physician who performs or orders the treatment or procedure is personally responsible for ensuring and certifying in the record that the informed consent process has taken place and that the patient has consented to the treatment or procedure. Exceptions to this include where informed consent is not possible without a serious threat to life or limb or if legally authorized by a court or judge.

(continued on page 97)

Figure 4-10. Minnesota Alliance for Patient Safety (MAPS) Template for Informed Consent Policy (continued)

The responsible physician is the physician performing the procedure. However, in cases where other practitioners actually perform the procedure it is the physician that supervises or orders the procedure.

A physician may collaborate with other practitioners who assist in the informed consent process or use patient education tools (i.e., video, written information sheets); however, it is the ordering, administering, or supervising physician that is responsible for obtaining the patient's informed consent and certifying that the process has occurred.

Facility's Responsibility
For procedures requiring written informed consent, the facility must assure the patient's right to make informed decisions by requiring practitioner(s) responsible for the surgery to obtain informed consent in a manner consistent with the policies governing the facility's informed consent process. The consent form is often provided by the facility and signed by the clinician and patient; however, the process may be initiated in the outpatient setting using a standardized form. For procedures requiring written informed consent, the facility must verify that written informed consent is in the patient's record before permitting the procedure to be performed.

Scope of Informed Consent
The scope of a patient's consent depends on what the clinician has discussed and what the patient has consented to. The scope of consent must be clear. It is important that the clinician explains and the patient understands the scope of what is being recommended, that both the clinician and patient are clear as to what the patient has consented to, and that their understanding is clearly documented on the informed consent form or elsewhere in the record.

A patient may consent to a one-time treatment or procedure (e.g., colonoscopy), routine care of a particular condition that may include a variety of discrete procedures or treatments (e.g., pre-natal care), or for a series of the same treatment (e.g., dialysis or blood transfusions during a hospital stay).

The patient can rescind consent at any time, especially when the scope covers several encounters.

PROCEDURES THAT MAY REQUIRE MORE THAN ONE CONSENT FORM

Sometimes several discrete procedures are ordered and administered by more than one physician (e.g., anesthesia before surgery, blood transfusion not related to surgery). In such a case, clinicians may obtain the patient's consent to the respective procedures on a single form.

If a single form is used, each clinician's signature certifies that the pertinent information for each procedure was discussed with the patient. If the form clearly identifies the procedures being consented to and is signed by both clinicians, facilities may use a different form for each procedure or treatment.

However, given that surgical procedures generally entail use of anesthesia, hospitals may wish to consider specifically extending their informed consent policies to include obtaining informed consent for the anesthesia component of the surgical procedure.

The informed consent form for surgery or invasive procedures does not include necessary informed consent required for research.

When Written Informed Consent IS Required
"Surgery" includes any procedure that is listed as a surgical procedure in the various billing or coding systems used by CMS or the hospitals, (e.g., CPT) regardless of whether Medicare pays for that surgical procedure.

(continued on page 98)

Figure 4-10. Minnesota Alliance for Patient Safety (MAPS) Template for Informed Consent Policy (continued)

Facility policy should specify which procedures are considered surgery and therefore are those that require a properly executed informed consent form. Medical staff by-laws should address which procedures and treatments require written informed consent

1. While a clinician should always communicate and collaborate with the patient regarding the patient's health care, federal and state law, rules of accrediting organizations and similar regulatory bodies require written informed consent for the following procedures:
    A. Surgical procedures (not including simple laceration repair and minor dermatological procedures performed in out-patient settings);
    B. Experimental procedures or treatment;
    C. Abortion;
    D. Administration of blood or blood products (if not related to the surgery/invasive procedure);
    E. Electro-convulsive therapy (ECT);
    F. Neuroleptic medication when prescribed for the treatment of mental illness or mental retardation (see policy on neuroleptic medication), but not when prescribed for other purposes;
    G. Any medical treatment necessary to preserve the life or health of a patient committed under the Minnesota Civil Commitment and Treatment Act;
    H. Radiation therapy;
    I. Invasive medical imaging;
    J. Procedures involving moderate to deep sedation where there is a risk of loss of protective reflexes (a separate anesthesia-specific consent form should be considered);
    K. Surgical or other invasive procedures involving a skin incision or puncture including, but not limited to: open surgical procedures, percutaneous aspiration, selected injections, biopsy, percutaneous cardiac and vascular diagnostic or interventional procedures, laparoscopies, endoscopies, and excluding venipuncture or intravenous therapy. Specific examples of other invasive procedures that require written informed consent are as follows:
        · Injections of any substance into a joint space or body cavity;
        · Percutaneous aspiration of body fluids through the skin (e.g., arthrocentesis, bone marrow aspiration, lumbar puncture, paracentesis, thoracentesis, suprapubic catheterization);
        · Biopsy (e.g., breast, liver, muscle, kidney, genitourinary, prostate, bladder, skin);
        · Cardiac procedures (e.g., cardiac catheterization, cardiac pacemaker implantation, angioplasty, stent implantation, intra-aortic balloon catheter insertion);
        · Central vascular access device insertion (e.g., Swan-Ganz catheter, percutaneous intravascular catheter (PIC) line, Hickman catheter);
        · Electrocautery of skin lesion;
        · Endoscopy (e.g., colonoscopy, bronchoscopy, esophagogastric endoscopy, cystoscopy, Percutaneous Endoscopic Gastrostomy (PEG), and J-tube placements, nephrostomy tube placements);
        · Laparoscopic surgical procedures (e.g., laparoscopic cholecystectomy, laparoscopic nephrectomy);
        · Invasive radiology procedures (e.g., angiography, angioplasty, percutaneous biopsy);
        · Laser therapy (e.g., eye, ear, nose, and throat (ENT));
        · Dermatology procedures (biopsy, excision and deep cryotherapy for malignant lesions - excluding cryotherapy for benign lesions);
        · Invasive ophthalmic procedures, including miscellaneous procedures involving implants;
        · Oral surgical procedures including tooth extraction and gingival biopsy;
        · Podiatric invasive procedures (removal of ingrown toenail, etc.);
        · Skin or wound debridement performed in an operating room; and
        · Renal dialysis.
    L. Diagnostic procedures that carry a significant, material risk;

(continued on page 99)

Figure 4-10. Minnesota Alliance for Patient Safety (MAPS) Template for Informed Consent Policy (continued)

    M. Circumcision;

    N. Sterilization;

    O. Continuation of a do-not-resuscitate or -intubate order (DNR or DNI) during surgery if the patient has a DNR or DNI order in place.

Exceptions to Informed Consent Requirement

The facility may permit a clinician to provide or order treatment without the patient's informed consent under two circumstances.

1. Emergencies. If an emergency medical condition makes it impossible or impractical to obtain informed consent without jeopardizing the patient's life or health, emergency treatment may be provided to preserve the patient's life or health. The emergency exception does not apply if the patient has previously clearly made known that he or she does not wish to receive the proposed emergency treatment under the present circumstances. The facts that make the situation an emergency must be documented in the patient's medical record. Emergency treatment under this exception may continue until the patient gains decision-making capacity, or until the patient's family or legal representative is available to make decisions on the patient's behalf, at which time informed consent must be obtained from the patient or the patient's representative.

2. Court-ordered treatment. Treatment may be provided to an individual without the individual's informed consent and over the patient's objection if ordered by a court. The court's order authorizing treatment must be documented in the patient's record.

TIMELINESS OF INFORMED CONSENT

1. The clinician must obtain the patient's informed consent before the procedure is administered, at a time that the patient is not sedated, and when the patient's judgment is not otherwise impaired.

2. If there is a delay between when the patient initially consented and when the procedure is performed, the patient's consent remains valid unless:
   A. There has been a significant deviation from the treatment plan to which the patient originally consented, in which case the patient must be informed of and consent to the change in plans; or
   B. Facts have changed since the clinician's discussion with the patient such that it would be reasonable for the patient to be informed of the change and asked to consent again in light of the changed facts, in which case the patient must be informed of the new facts and be asked consent in light of them; or
   C. The patient has revoked consent, in which case the procedure may not be performed.

Even if there has been no significant change, a clinician should discuss the proposed treatment with the patient again if more than 30 days have passed between the initial discussion and consent and the day that the procedure will be administered. It is not necessary to sign a new consent form if the clinician documents the discussion in the patient's record.

WHO CAN GIVE INFORMED CONSENT

1. Patient with decision-making capacity: A patient with decision-making capacity is the only person who may consent to his or her own treatment. While the patient may include and consult with others in the patient's decision-making process, the clinician must not proceed with the procedure unless the patient consents. In general, a person lacks capacity if the person (1) does not demonstrate a general awareness of his or her health situation and the treatment being proposed; (2) cannot understand the factual information provided about the recommended treatment, especially its risks and benefits; or (3) cannot communicate – verbally or nonverbally

(continued on page 100)

Figure 4-10. Minnesota Alliance for Patient Safety (MAPS) Template for Informed Consent Policy (continued)

– a clear decision regarding the treatment based on that information.

The clinician should assess the patient's capacity each time the patient is asked to consent to a procedure. If the clinician determines that the patient lacks capacity to give or withhold consent, the facts supporting that determination must be documented in the patient's medical record.

2. Adults: In general, an adult age 18 or over is presumed to have decision-making capacity unless there is convincing evidence to the contrary. If a clinician concludes that a patient lacks capacity, he or she should note in a patient's record the facts and reasons supporting that decision. This presumption does not apply if the person has been found by a court to currently have diminished decision-making capacity; for example, a person whose court-appointed guardian has been given the power to make medical decisions.

Disagreement with the recommendation of a health-care professional is not evidence of incapacity.

3. A patient without decision-making capacity: If a patient lacks decision-making capacity, informed consent must be obtained from a representative of the patient. The first person on the following list who is available and willing to serve may be recognized as the patient's representative:
    A. A parent or guardian if the patient is a child age 17 or younger;
    B. A court-appointed guardian with authority to make health care decisions for the patient;
    C. A health-care agent named by the patient in a health-care directive, health-care power of attorney, or similar document; or
    D. A friend or relative of the patient who knows the patient well enough to know what the patient would decide if they had the capacity and who is willing to make decisions on the patient's behalf.

    NOTE: Except for patients being treated under the Minnesota Civil Commitment and Treatment Act, there is no prescribed order or hierarchy of relatives or friends who may act as the patient's representative. Depending on the circumstances, the representative may be the patient's spouse, life partner or companion, parent, adult child, neighbor, friend, or other person. The only necessary criterion is that the person know the patient well enough to be able to state with reasonable confidence what the patient would likely decide if the patient were able to do so.

    The clinician should consider the patient's representative to be the person who best knows the patient and what the patient would likely decide if the patient had capacity, and who will make decisions in accord with the patient's wishes. The hospital and clinic may assist the clinician in making this determination.

4. Joint decision-makers: More than one person may serve as the patient's representative. For example, a patient's health-care directive may name two or more persons to act jointly as the patient's agent, or two adult children may act jointly as the representative for their incapacitated parent. If more than one potential representative is available and they cannot agree to act jointly, the clinician may decide who among the potential decision-makers will most likely make the decisions the patient would make and designate that person as the patient's representative for purposes of obtaining informed consent. The clinician is required to document the process by which the representative is determined.

The patient's representative should be asked whether the patient would have consented to the proposed treatment if the patient were capable of making the decision. If it is impossible to know what the patient would have chosen, the representative may make the decision based on what is in the patient's best interest. The clinician should document in the patient's medical record the process used to determine who will be the decision-maker and the reasons for the clinician's determination.

(continued on page 101)

Figure 4-10. Minnesota Alliance for Patient Safety (MAPS) Template for Informed Consent Policy (continued)

5. Children: A person younger than 18 years is presumed not to have legal capacity to make health care decisions and a parent or guardian must make health-care decisions for the child. However, a child younger than 18 years has legal capacity to give informed consent without the consent of anyone else in the following circumstances:
   A. A person age 17 or younger may give (or withhold) informed consent to any medical care if the person:
      - has borne a child; or
      - is married; or
      - lives apart from his or her parents or guardians and is managing his or her own financial affairs. The source or amount of the minor's income is not relevant.
   B. Any person who is 17 or younger may give (or withhold) informed consent for treatment related to:
      - pregnancy (including birth control) or sexually transmitted disease; or
      - drug or alcohol dependency; or
      - admission for mental illness or chemical dependency, but only if an examiner determines that the child has mental illness or chemical dependency and is suitable for treatment.

   A parent's consent to treatment does not impose an obligation on the clinician to provide it.

Tania Daniels, Vice President, Patient Safety
Minnesota Hospital Association
2550 University Ave. W., Suite 350-S
Saint Paul, MN 55114-1900
(800) 462-5393 or (651) 641-1121
tdaniels@mnhospitals.org

form cover all the things that are in here or not? Is ours readable at the fifth- or sixth-grade level?' There's no requirement that you have to actually follow the template exactly. It's just a best practice." For example, HealthEast's final version of the template calls the form a "Verification of Informed Consent for Surgery or Invasive Procedures," emphasizing that the form is the last step in the overall process.

MAPS soon plans to do a full survey of Minnesota hospitals, systems, and surgery centers to find out how many are using the informed consent templates.

The standardization of the form and policy took approximately a year and a half, and translation of the form into different languages began in 2008. The MHLP, which is a program of the Minnesota Literacy Council that promotes health literacy across the state, assisted with the process. "We have translated the consent form into Spanish, Russian, and Somali," notes Lane Stiles, director, Fairview Press, and MHLP's representative on the MAPS work group. "The English version is on one half of the page, and the translation on the other, so the physician and the patient are always looking at the same thing." Although professional translators are currently working on other languages as well, Stiles warns against the misconception that limited English or reading skills are the only determinants to health literacy: "People think it is simply limited English proficiency or they reduce it down to functional literacy issues. The real problem is communication. That takes two people, and the burden is on us to take patients as they come and communicate according to what they need. We advocate universal precautions because [health literacy] is almost impossible to assess. Anybody at any time, no matter how you might assess by different scales, can be health illiterate for any physical, mental, or emotional reason."

Daniels agrees that observing universal precautions—making all materials easy for everyone to understand—is a best practice: "The goal is to create a standard across the state so that no matter which facility patients or providers are at, they are familiar with the MAPS consent process and form."

In March 2008 the MMA targeted physicians, particularly those who perform inpatient and outpatient procedures, for dissemination of the new consent form and policy. The association sent out an e-mail describing the communitywide process; assuring members that it met all regulatory requirements; and stressing that the new form could improve office efficiency, streamline processes, and minimize work for staff. Some physicians were initially uncertain about their role and responsibilities in the informed consent process, and a few clinics asked permission to make minor adjustments to the language to adapt it to their practices; however, overall implementation has gone well.

Adding Scope

To further its goal to assist patients in participating effectively in their own care, MAPS also developed a medication reconciliation guide to help them keep track of their allergies, the medications they are currently taking and have taken, why they were prescribed, by whom, and any side effects that occurred. Twenty-three MAPS member organizations partnered on this project, which began in 2006, along with AARP and the state's home care association and board of social workers. The development process followed the same lines as that for the informed consent policy and form, with the group using existing reconciliation forms as a starting point, meeting to discuss necessary changes, and distributing different versions among group members for feedback. The University of Minnesota's Academic Health Center helped to distribute the final version of *My Medicine List* (*see* Figure 4-11, page 103) at the Minnesota State Fair in 2006, and both the tool and an explanatory brochure are available online (http://www.mnpatientsafety.org). The English version of the medicine list is available in different font sizes, and it has been translated into several languages, including Spanish, Russian, Somali, and Vietnamese.

Building Relationships and Support

The process of developing tools and promoting health literacy has shown participants where challenges are likely to occur and how to address them. For example, many leaders and health care professionals are unaware of the extent or impact of poor health literacy,

Figure 4-11. *My Medicine List* for Patients

Medication Tracking Form
Fold this form and keep it with you

Name:	Date of Birth:	**Allergic To:** *(Describe reaction)*
Emergency Contact/Phone numbers:		
Doctor(s):		
Pharmacies, other sources:		

Immunization Record *(Record the date/year of last dose taken)*		Flu vaccine(s):		
Pneumonia vaccine:	Tetanus:	Hepatitis vaccine:	Other: (type) date:	

List all medicines you are currently taking. Include prescriptions (examples: pills, inhalers, creams, shots), over-the-counter medications (examples: aspirin, antacids, vitamins) and herbals (examples: ginseng, gingko). Include medications taken as needed (example: nitroglycerin, inhalers).

START DATE	NAME OF MEDICATION	DOSE	DIRECTIONS *(How do you take it? When? How often?)*	DATE STOPPED	NOTES *(Reason for taking?)*

Directions

1. ALWAYS KEEP THIS FORM WITH YOU. You may want to fold it and keep it in your wallet along with your driver's license. Then it will be available in case of an emergency.

2. Write down all of the medicines you are taking and list all of your allergies. Add information on medicines taken in clinics, hospitals and other health care settings — as well as at home.

3. Take this form with you on all visits to your clinic, pharmacy, hospital, physician, or other providers.

4. WRITE DOWN ALL CHANGES MADE TO YOUR MEDICINES on this form. When you stop taking a certain medicine, write the date it was stopped. If help is needed, ask your doctor, nurse, pharmacist, or family member to help you keep it up-to-date.

5. In the "Notes" column, write down why you are taking the medicine (Examples: high blood pressure, high blood sugar, high cholesterol).

6. When you are discharged from the hospital, someone will talk with you about which medicines to take and which medicines to stop taking. Since many changes are often made after a hospital stay, a new list may be filled out. When you return to your doctor, take your list with you. This will keep everyone up-to-date on your medicines.

How does this form help you?

- This form helps you and your family members remember all of the medicines you are taking. If appropriate, consider sharing your information with adult children.

- It provides your doctors and other providers with a current list of ALL of your medicines. They need to know the herbals, vitamins, and over-the-counter medicines you take!

- With this information, doctors and other providers can prevent potential health problems, triggered by how different medicines interact.

 For copies of the medication tracking form and a brochure with more tips, visit the Minnesota Alliance for Patient Safety's Web site at www.mnpatientsafety.org or call (651) 641-1121; toll free (800) 462-5393.

Source: Used with permission of the Minnesota Alliance for Patient Safety.

This form, which was developed based on best practices for medication reconciliation, is available online for patients' use. The form can be printed out and filled in so the patient can carry it with him or her to each physician appointment. This type of form is particularly useful for avoiding polypharmacy issues with geriatric patients and others who see multiple specialists and take multiple medications.

and it can be difficult to overcome that apathy. "Try to decide how you'd make a business case for this when you take it to senior leadership and where your partners might be in the organization," advises Stiles. "Patient safety is certainly a big driver now, and that's one way to quickly get senior leadership on board. But there are clinical quality, compliance, and patient satisfaction issues as well. When you start breaking this down, there are a lot of different parts to the health care system that have a vested interest in health literacy even if they don't know it. There are a lot of different people who will be partners if you try to implement practical reforms in your system."

Moravec suggests bringing up the point of legal responsibility: "Consider the ramifications of *not* communicating well, whether it's a consent form or a discharge process that people don't understand. Look at the consent form you have and try it out with some of your staff and patients in a pilot or focus group. You'll probably find a lot of the patients who will say, 'We don't understand it. We just sign it.' And your legal department will tell you you're not protected even though you have a signed consent form. A consent form that is unreadable is not a protection." To get the word out to other physicians, he has talked about health literacy and the MAPS templates during grand rounds; in lectures for nursing staff and presentations to surgeons' committees; and in discussions with residents, medical staff leadership, and executives. He has also written articles for HealthEast's medical staff newsletter, some of which have been picked up by the MMA's journal as well.

Taking your audience's concerns into account is also important when introducing changes in communication methods and policies. "We push patients through our systems much faster than we did 20 years ago," notes Stiles. "When you compress time with patients, teaching and communication time is often squeezed out. That's a problem we have to address. Part of this is how we reintegrate communication into clinical workflows, how we bring back time for clinicians to interact and communicate. There are a lot of challenges and no simple solutions."

Including patient representatives and advocates in both development and presentation to staff can be extremely helpful. Getting up-front input from patients can help other team members understand the needs of the real "end users" of the forms and processes they're revising and save rework when pilot tests of more difficult materials prove unsuccessful. Giving patients a voice also gives them a sense of ownership, encouraging them to participate more fully in their own care. "People were very respectful, and I felt that I was listened to at all the meetings," says Norton of her experiences on the MAPS work group. "I think it's truly important for an advocate not only to be there in name but to make an effort to learn about the topic and contribute. I never felt like a token member of the group."

Putting the emphasis on patients is the foundation for any health literacy effort. "My mantra is 'Look at the patient,'" says Stiles. "If what you're doing isn't benefitting patient in some way and putting the patient first, stop and think of another way to do it."

CASE STUDY: NEW YORK UNIVERSITY SCHOOL OF MEDICINE/BELLEVUE HOSPITAL CENTER

Medication errors are one of the most common problems throughout health care, and children are an particularly vulnerable population. Health literacy is a major factor when parents and other caregivers try to administer medications in the home, because misunderstandings about what constitutes the proper dosage, when each dose should be given, and how long the medication regimen should continue frequently contribute to errors. In an effort to reduce these types of mistakes, staff at the New York University School of Medicine (NYUSOM)/Bellevue Hospital Center developed a new strategy to improve the way medication information is presented to parents that includes patient-specific instruction sheets with pictograms and teach-back as part of medication counseling.

Bellevue is an 800-bed public hospital serving the four boroughs of New York City. The flagship hospital of the New York City Health and Hospitals Corporation (HHC), it has more than 450,000 clinic visits and approximately 90,000 emergency department (ED) visits a year, with about 65,000 and 20,000 of them, respectively, in pediatrics. The hospital is closely affiliated with NYUSOM. About 68% of the pediatric patient population is Hispanic, 16% is Asian, and 15% is African American. Approximately 40% are recent immigrants with limited English proficiency. Most of the pediatric patient population are from low-income families who depend on Medicaid (60%) or Child Health Plus, New York State's health insurance for children (25%); 13% is uninsured. Addressing the health literacy of parents is a priority in both the pediatric clinic and the pediatric ED.

Identifying a Need

Seven years ago, Bellevue introduced a program called the Health Education and Literacy for Parents (HELP) Project, which grew out of the hospital's participation in Reach Out and Read, a national early literacy

intervention. Recognizing that any efforts aimed at children's literacy needs must also address the needs of their parents, HELP staff and trained volunteers conduct short-term educational activities with parents in pediatric waiting rooms. The activities, which may be one-on-one or in small groups, offer strategies to help parents improve their families' health and pursue their own education. The volunteers are mainly multilingual NYU premedicine students, who undergo extensive training to learn how to help parents understand how to perform health-related tasks such as reading prescription labels and asking their physician questions about their child's health. "While working with parents in the HELP Project, it became clear that there was a tremendous amount of parental confusion about how to administer medicines," recalls Linda van Schaick, M.S.Ed., founder and director of the HELP Project. "The final impetus for developing the medication instruction sheet intervention occurred when I saw a family leaving the clinic after their pediatrician's visit. The mom was holding a paper towel with a picture of a syringe on it, drawn by their physician to show how much medicine to use. I realized we could really do a lot better than that. We started looking at how to create an intervention that would be specific to the individual patient's prescription, use plain language and pictures, and be available in the family's language."

While confusion about medications included issues such as lack of understanding about what medicines were supposed to do and why they should be continued for a certain length of time, confusion about dosing instruments was also a significant issue. Manufacturers market many different kinds of instruments, including dosing spoons, dosing cups, droppers, and oral dosing syringes. All are considered standardized because they have been created to measure specific amounts, as opposed to teaspoons and tablespoons, which can vary greatly in actual quantity. "When we first started this project, we thought parents must be getting a dosing instrument to measure medications from the pharmacy," says van Schaick. "When we realized that many were not getting any dosing tools, it became clear why they were reaching for nonstandardized spoons."

Even when instruments are made available for parents, the variation between and within instrument types can be baffling to users. "As health care providers, we often give very specific instructions," notes H. Shonna Yin, M.D., M.S., assistant professor of pediatrics at NYUSOM/Bellevue. "Pediatricians don't just give instructions in 5-milliliter increments; medication dosing for children is largely weight-based, and doses as specific as 1.2 or 3.5 milliliters may be prescribed. In addition to this, some dosing instruments contain markings that add unnecessary complexity—for example, dosing instruments with markings given in 0.4- or 0.625-milliliter increments. These are systems barriers that should be addressed to decrease the literacy demands placed on families."

To counteract these problems, the HELP Project staff began work on the HELPix intervention in 2003. They started with the development of medication instruction sheets that parents could take home and use for reference during the duration of a child's drug regimen, then moved on to revise the way counseling was provided during the patient encounter.

Creating Instruction Sheets

Existing materials used in providing medical care in nonliterate cultures provided a starting point for staff, and it was here that van Schaick first saw pictograms. The United States Pharmacopeia (USP) pictogram library provided the next source, but it was not optimal given the focus on adult rather than pediatric patients. "In pediatrics, there is a reliance on liquid formulations of medicines, particularly for young children, and this is closely linked to the issue of standardized dosing instrument use. The USP pictograms were not designed to address this issue," says Yin. In the end, it was necessary to develop new pictograms. A part-time staff member from the Child Development Department who was also a graphic artist was tapped to create the pictograms, and

the HELPix project got special funding to allow her to work on them. (Now retired, she is still an outside consultant for the project.)

In addition to designing the medication instruction sheets themselves, it was necessary to develop a procedure to generate the sheets. The initial attempt involved a fill-in PDF template that physicians could access from the clinic's desktop computers. Staff realized that hundreds of different PDFs would be required to account for the large number of different medicines, indications, doses, instructions related to dosing frequency, length of treatment, and languages. A software prototype was pilot tested to address this need and was used as part of a randomized control trial to evaluate the efficacy of the intervention based on the medication instruction sheets. "Initially, the pediatricians had to shade in an empty syringe that was not a standard 5- or 10-milliliter dose to the right point," says van Schaick. "With the first software prototype, the exact color and proportion were automatically shown in the pictogram for every prescription written. The flexibility of the prototype allowed us to generate instruction sheets for more medications and a larger variety of treatment regimens."

To use the software application, physicians first select a medicine from a drop-down menu. Based on that selection, a list of available formulations (such as tablets, caplets, or geltabs) is shown, followed by a choice of different strengths. Physicians then indicate the specifics of the prescribed medication regimen. Based on this information, the database applies the appropriate instructions and pictograms to the handout, which is then printed out for the parents. "The information entered is a little redundant," admits Yin. "Our hospital has electronic medication prescribing, so when the physicians are writing their prescriptions, they will be entering a lot of the same information into the program. We had originally hoped to link the software to our electronic prescribing system so the physicians wouldn't have to do double work, but this wasn't possible. So we are developing the software as a stand-alone application with the hope of someday being able to connect it with electronic prescribing systems." There have been some benefits to the software being a separate entity: van

Figure 4-12. HELPix Instruction Sheet for an Antibiotic

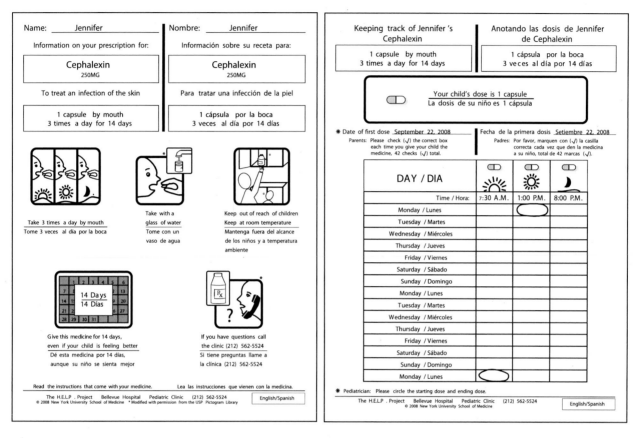

Source: Used with permission of New York University School of Medicine.

Instructions for a patient's specific prescription include the drug name, amount and frequency of dose, duration of regimen, what the medication looks like, and how it should be administered. The physician circles the beginning and ending doses on the daily log; parents check off the appropriate box after each dose is given.

Schaick and Yin have been approached by other facilities that use different electronic prescribing systems or do not have electronic prescribing but would be able to use a Web-based application. Yin notes that having the application accessible on the Internet has significant implications for dissemination.

The project began with a focus on liquid medicines—first daily-dose medications such as antibiotics, and then nonprescription or as-needed drugs such as acetaminophen, ibuprofen, and diphenhydramine. The daily-dose and as-needed medications required slightly different handouts. Daily-dose medications came with log sheets for parents to fill out as they gave each dose;

this ensured that doses were not forgotten and that the entire prescription was used. As-needed medication sheets reinforced the concept that medicines should be administered as required by symptoms and included a special log that helped parents ensure that the maximum number of allowable doses per day was not exceeded. Medications in pill form have since been added to the available options.

The instruction sheets are either bilingual (*see* Figure 4-12, above) or monolingual in English and Spanish. Plans are currently underway to add other languages, such as Bengali, French, and Chinese, as soon as possible.

Conducting a Randomized Trial

In 2006, after the initial instruction sheets for liquid medications had been developed, NYUSOM/Bellevue decided to conduct a randomized control trial to test the efficacy of the handouts. Staff recognized that they needed a standardized intervention that included an improved counseling process as well as visual aids. "Traditional counseling was generally verbal counseling given by the child's physician," explains Yin. "In our ED, parents also received postconferencing from a nurse before going home, so medications were reviewed twice. Most of the time there was no standard handout; the provider could give them something printed from an online source like Medline, but it was not specific to a patient's regimen. And it was up to each physician whether a dosing instrument was provided or teach-back was used."

For the trial, which took place in Bellevue's pediatric ED from July through December 2006, families were randomized to receive either the pictogram- based instruction sheets or routine counseling. For those who received the intervention, trained research assistants printed out the appropriate sheets and used them to guide medication counseling. Counseling, which was provided at discharge, also included demonstration of the dosing procedure by the research assistant, as well as teach-back and show-back by parents (having parents demonstrate how they would measure a dose using the dosing instrument), provision of the standardized dosing instrument, and a walk-through of the medication log. Families who were recruited from the ED waiting room to participate were assessed for sociodemographic characteristics, the child's medical history, and the parent's/ caregiver's health literacy level (using the Test of Functional Health Literacy in Adults). Follow-up assessments—which addressed knowledge of medication, related behaviors (such as storage method) dosing frequency, and adherence (for daily-dose drugs)—were conducted in person and/or by phone. Families were targeted for follow-up beginning either three to five days after their ED visits, for as-needed medications, or within one day of the expected end of a daily-dose regimen. The overall results showed that parents who received the new intervention exhibited much better dosing accuracy and adherence to medication regimens.*

"From what we saw in the study, the intervention worked very well," says Yin. "While some providers have raised concerns about whether the pictogram-based intervention would add significant additional time to the medication counseling process, we did not find that to be the case in the trial. Using the intervention provides structure to the counseling process, making the process more effective and efficient."

Building Support

Much of the success of the HELPix project can be traced to the interest and support that NYUSOM/Bellevue clinicians and staff contributed throughout the process. "Our clinic medical directors have been very supportive of our work," states van Schaick. "And the clinic physicians have been incredibly helpful in giving me their perspectives. In addition, other clinic staff members have provided invaluable linguistic and cultural perspectives to the development of the intervention. They've given an enormous amount of their time and feedback. It's been a tribute to how much they really care about these issues."

She sees the course of the project paralleling the growing interest in health literacy in the health care field. Whereas people did not fully understand the issue of health literacy in the beginning, there is now a strong interest, particularly within the organization's leadership. Yin agrees: "As people have heard about the HELPix intervention and our research findings, there has been a lot of excitement from the physicians and nurses in the pediatric clinic and ED about having this intervention available for use in patient care."

Outside partners have also been valuable. The New York City Poison Control Center, which is located across the street from Bellevue, started a health literacy program for LEP learners in adult education called

---

* Yin H.S., et al.: Randomized control trial of a pictogram-based intervention to reduce liquid medication dosing errors and improve adherence among caregivers of young children. *Arch Pediatr Adolesc Med* 162:814–822, Sep. 2008.

HELP at the same time the hospital began its HELP Project. Pharmacists at the Poison Control Center have been able to provide a crucial perspective, addressing questions about how drugs should be administered and which warnings are most important. They critically reviewed the pictograms and instructions on the HELPix instruction sheets to be sure each made sense.

Parents have also been an important part of the process, giving feedback during ongoing pilot testing. "If we needed a pictogram to show something like 'wait four hours before giving another dose of this medicine,' we had our graphic designer draw three or four ways of showing that. Then we would go to different language and cultural groups within our clinic and present the different pictures with the words underneath them to see whether there was any consensus on which picture made the most sense to our audience," explains van Schaick. "We have also embedded pilot testing within the HELP Project itself. We found that parents were really disarmed when we said we needed their help and their opinion, and they gave us a lot of input. We took many of their suggestions; they really felt that their opinions were valued."

Parents were particularly vocal about pictograms and instructions pertaining to dosing instruments. "The pictogram that parents use and like the most is the dosing diagram, because it visually shows them how much medication to use within a specific instrument," says Yin. Because as-needed medicines such as infant acetaminophen and ibuprofen have their own instruments, specific pictograms depicting doses with those instruments were created. According to van Schaick, "Sometimes parents were given instructions for a medication that would say '1 dropper full.' They would think that this meant to fill the whole dropper, which makes sense. But physicians may actually mean to the highest line, and sometimes there is still a significant amount of the dropper that should be left empty. So we began to realize how truly necessary it was to give people a visual reinforcement of *exactly* what they should measure out as their child's dose." (*See* Figure 4-13, page 110.)

Funding for both the development of the instruc-

tion sheets and the research study have been provided by different sources from both inside and outside NYUSOM/Bellevue—including the HHC, Altman, and United Hospital Fund Foundations—over the years.

Taking the Next Step

Although the combination of pictogram-based medication instruction sheets and teach-back as part of medication counseling has proven to be efficacious in the pediatric ED, leaders at NYUSOM/Bellevue now want to determine whether the intervention will work in a clinical setting when used by physicians as part of routine medication counseling. To this end, a pre-postimplementation study has been initiated in Bellevue Hospital's pediatric outpatient clinic. "We've already finished gathering the baseline data, so we have a sense of how well parents in our clinic are doing with medication dosing and adherence," explains Yin. "Once we complete the Web-based application, we'll train all the physicians, make the application accessible from the desktop computers in each patient room, and see how physicians use it. We'll be talking to parents to see how they feel about the intervention and whether their pediatrician performed the different parts of the intervention." One of the questions the study will address is whether dosing accuracy and other measures will be altered if a physician does not include all the steps of the intervention (for example, skipping teach-back or show-back, or not providing a standardized dosing instrument).

Yin and van Schaick, who will be training the physicians for the trial, want to build on the existing interest in the instruction sheets that the pediatrics staff has shown. According to Yin, "We want to generate a lot of excitement so that physicians will be motivated to use the intervention, because we recognize that it will add another step that they will have to do as part of their routine. We will emphasize that the HELPix intervention does not really take any extra time compared to their traditional counseling; it is meant to be a strategy that will allow for more efficient and effective counseling. As part of the provider training module, we are going to emphasize the issue of health literacy and the high rate of errors we've found in the clinic and the ED."

Figure 4-13. HELPix Instruction Sheet for As-Needed Medication

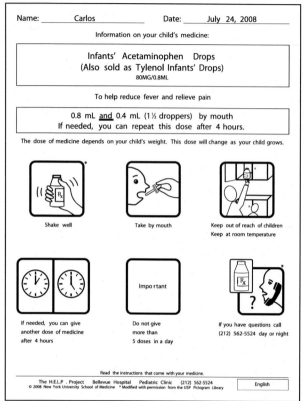
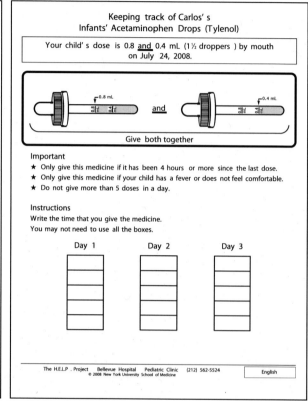

Source: Used with permission of New York University School of Medicine.

Handouts like this one give the exact dose required in words and numbers, as well as in a drawing that matches the dropper given with the acetaminophen drops so parents can be sure they are administering the correct amount.

Getting physician buy-in also depends on giving them a sense of ownership over the process, including involving them in the adaptation and refinement of the intervention. "We want to find out what the physicians feel are the barriers and try to address them," says van Schaick. "We want them to feel that we're being responsive to their feedback."

Planning for the Future

As they test the instruction sheets for medications in liquid and pill form in the outpatient clinic, the staff plan to develop handouts for other medication forms such as sprays, topicals, and inhalers. They are also currently working on creating plain-language, photograph-based medication instruction sheets to help

parents manage their children's asthma medicine. As van Schaick notes, "We're learning and adapting things all the time. The instruction sheets are definitely a work in progress."

Significant potential exists to adapt the HELPix intervention to other settings and populations. For example, the pharmacy is typically the final point where families might receive medication counseling, and it is the site where final decisions on strength and dose may be changed from a physician's original instructions. "Many studies have shown that pharmacists often don't provide counseling," says Yin. "Use of the HELPix intervention at the pharmacy level would serve to reinforce the medication instructions given by providers." Van

Schaick agrees: "It would be interesting to do a pilot study at the pharmacy and see how our sheets could be used there."

Health care professionals who work in geriatrics and have seen the instruction sheets are also enthusiastic about the potential for adapting them to this population. The elderly are at high risk for limited health literacy and medication errors. However, several major considerations would need to be addressed before the pediatric tools could be adapted for adults. For example, adults tend to take medicines on an ongoing basis rather than over a short course. Most older adults also take multiple medications, so developers would need to figure out a way to combine instructions and daily logs for each patient rather than giving out separate sheets for each drug.

The journey from designing the first pictograms to establishing a usable software application and comprehensive intervention has been an iterative process that has taken almost five years. When more testing has been completed and adjustments made, the goal is to make the intervention available to other facilities. "The Web-based application is a dream come true," says van Schaick. "We now have the potential to improve parent understanding of medication instructions at many more pediatric health facilities."

CASE STUDY: LUTHERAN HEALTHCARE

Trying to evaluate and monitor the literacy level of patient materials across a large health system can be a daunting task. The sheer number of educational and promotional brochures, forms, and other print pieces generated by different departments makes ensuring consistency a problem—one you may not realize you have until something brings it to your attention. This was the case for Lutheran HealthCare—a system that includes Lutheran Medical Center; 8 Lutheran Family Health Center sites; the Lutheran Augustana Center for Extended Care and Rehabilitation; 14 school-based clinics; 3 senior housing facilities; Health Plus, a managed Medicaid program; and widespread community support programs: all based in Brooklyn, New York. The system's many components serve a diverse area that includes Arabic, Chinese, Hispanic, Orthodox Jewish, and Russian populations, and 24% of local residents live below the federal poverty level.

Recognizing a Need

It was when staff tried to identify and prioritize forms for translation that questions regarding readability started to surface. "We realized that in an effort to turn things around quickly using limited resources we had been putting the cart before the horse," says Virginia Tong, M.S.W., vice president of Cultural Competence. "Translation should really be the final step when making a document patient-ready. We had to figure out what needed to be addressed first and how to get those processes in place and hardwired into a large and complicated system. We realized we were wasting resources; a lot of what we were translating remained unreadable because the literacy level was too high for our target audience."

The president and CEO of the health care system asked Karen Lennon, M.S., senior vice president of External Affairs, to "review all written patient materials and come up with a plan that would work quickly, effectively, and systemwide." The resulting group, aptly named the "Paper Chase" Committee, convened in 2006 and included a multidisciplinary group of representatives from the departments of adult education and training, cultural competence, marketing, and public relations. Their task was to perform a complete, systemic review of all patient print pieces; make recommendations to issuing departments on areas that needed improvement; and implement systemwide training.

The process began when departments across the system were instructed to create a binder of all documents they distributed to the general public and patient population. In reading through the approximately 30 binders that were submitted, the review committee found a host of inconsistencies that could be problematic for those who read at a sixth-grade level or below. "The reading level was too high," recalls Kathy Johannesen, M.P.A., marketing director. "There was missing information such as logos, addresses, and telephone numbers. Some sheets had been copied so many times that you couldn't make out half the words." There was also a great deal of technical language embedded in a large amount of text. "It was almost as though people were writing to professionals as opposed to the general community," says Kathleen Hopkins, director of Community-Based Programs. "The materials were primarily very dense word documents instead of easy-to-understand text complemented with graphics."

Translated documents also came under scrutiny, and several issues were identified. Many of the translations were of questionable quality because they had been done by people who were not fluent in the language. There were inconsistencies in how various terms were translated, even including the name of the organization or program. There also seemed to be no criteria for which documents were translated into which languages, and different translations of the same document were not done consistently.

In general, health system details were also an issue. The authors of each piece often included their own definition of their unit or site. For instance, one document might include some introductory language about the facility with a mission statement. "Although the writers had good intentions, the documents looked like they could have come from several different hospitals," notes Neal Gorman, vice president of public relations. "With everyone listing a different mission statement and defining 'who we are' in their own terms, it left our main core message very disjointed."

The committee developed a new policy and process by which all new materials and those to be revised or reprinted would be reviewed by external affairs and adult education staff, and then forwarded to the Cultural Competence department for translation. The new policy and procedure were introduced at the monthly systemwide department head meeting in May 2007. At that time, the committee presented "before and after" documents that clearly showed department heads the difference this process could make. "We had fun with the presentation, but the message was clear," recalls Lennon. "If your patient doesn't understand your message, you may not know until it is too late. Information such as how to take your medicine, when to call your doctor, and the next steps in your medical care must be carefully and clearly communicated."

Representatives from other areas were also brought into the project to create a system of checks and balances. The committee found that some documents were being sent for printing without any form of review, so the head of the system's print shop was asked to watch for these materials and forward them to the committee. In addition, Lennon became a member of the Lutheran HealthCare forms committee (which has to approve every form that is used in the medical record) to catch any pieces that had reached that committee without going through the health literacy/translation review.

Training the Authors

When the policy was rolled out, the review committee wanted to begin training those who created written pieces across the organization. The curriculum, developed by the Paper Chase Committee and the Organizational Learning Department (a division of human resources that facilitates staff education), was jump-started by returning each department's original submitted binder with committee suggestions attached. Trainers used those binders as a basis to discuss the new review process, literacy issues that should be considered in writing patient materials, and how those considerations could be put to use in the specific department. Training is now delivered by adult education staff once a quarter (*see* Figure 4-14, pages 114–115), although the committee would like to increase the frequency if additional resources can be found. A small pamphlet of things to remember and ways to work around such things as technical language is distributed to attendees for future reference (*see* Figure 4-15, page 115).

The review committee faced a certain amount of resistance from staff, who did not think the new process was necessary. "People don't have a very strong sense of how pervasive literacy issues are, so it doesn't occur to them that there might be people who don't read as well as they do," notes Stacie Evans, education coordinator. "They don't understand that they might have more education or experience with reading than some of the people who are going to read their document." To counteract this mind-set, the system held mandatory cultural competence training for all personnel, which included a 10-minute excerpt from the AMA Foundation health literacy video. The vignettes, showing English-speaking people who did not seem to be at risk of low health literacy but did not understand what hypertension was or how to take oral medications, were conversation starters; many staff were shocked that such problems existed.

Implementing the Policy

All patient education pieces are now sent through external affairs, but each department in the system has its own way of developing materials. For example, the rehabilitation staff write their own pieces, and review staff may only simplify the language. Other departments, such as cardiac care, may tell external affairs staff what they want, indicate sources to be used and points to be highlighted, and ask for the final product to be sent to them for approval. Many people in the system are not yet aware of the review policy or how to prepare reader-friendly products because they have not yet received

Figure 4-14. Agenda for Training In-House Writers

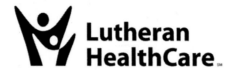

Writing Patient Materials:
Training Curriculum Agenda

I. Introduction
  A. Welcome
  B. Introduce training objectives
  C. Participants introduce themselves, including name, position/dept, experience writing patient materials, and goals for today.

II. Health Literacy Game Show
  A. Interactive quiz game involving true/false and multiple choice questions about health literacy. Prizes!

III. Hands-On Activity: Writing clear instructions for a mystery task
  A. Participants are divided into two groups; each group's task is hidden from the other. Each member of Group 1 is given a paper airplane, and must write instructions on how to build it. Each member of Group 2 is given a picture and must write instructions on how to draw it.
  B. Group 1 and 2 trade instructions. Each person tries to follow his/her instructions to accomplish that specific task.
  C. Reflect on the results and discuss the challenges of writing clear instructions.

IV. "Before and After" Examples
  A. Distribute copies of a confusing brochure that was written for patients at an inappropriately high literacy level.
  B. Divide into teams (small groups of about four people). Each team discusses the brochure's strengths and weaknesses as related to patient understanding. Each team then writes a list of specific ways in which they would suggest revising it.
  C. Distribute copies of the actual revised version of the brochure (two rack cards).
  D. The whole group now identifies what kinds of changes were made to the original brochure, and which team's list had the most relevant suggestions.

V. Guidelines for Writing Patient Materials
  A. Distribute copies of the *Writing Patient Materials* tip sheet. Allow time for participants to read through it and address any questions or concerns they may have. Also ask pilot participants to give us feedback on the presentation of the tip sheet (its format, length, usefulness, etc.).

(continued on page 115)

This plan shows the components of Lutheran HealthCare's training sessions to help staff create easy-to-read printed materials. In addition to conducting a "quiz show" to make participants aware of health literacy issues and presenting guidelines for good writing practices, the session includes hands-on activities so participants gain experience in applying those guidelines.

Figure 4-14. Agenda for Training In-House Writers (continued)

VI.   Hands-On Revision Process
A.   Each participant sits at a computer where they open, in Microsoft Word, a confusing document that was written for patients at an inappropriately high literacy level – specifically, this document addresses AFP screening for pregnant women. (A hard copy of the document is also distributed.)
B.   Participants work individually on revising the document – using the Writing Patient Materials tip sheet – to make it more patient-friendly.
C.   Using the projector, two or three participants' revised versions of the document are projected on the wall for the group to read and discuss.

VII.   Wrap-Up
A.   Participants share what they learned in this workshop and relate it to their original goals for the day. Time for any remaining questions.
B.   Facilitators explain the new protocol for all patient materials, including the process each document goes through and a rough timeframe for turnaround.

VIII.   Training Evaluation forms

Source: Lutheran HealthCare. Used with permission.

training. "One of the obstacles we come across in our system is the lack of availability in people's schedules to attend training, but we often connect with people when they ask to have a document translated or printed. That's when we bring them into the process, and because of the checks and balances we've created, very few can actually work outside the system," explains Hopkins.

When individual pieces are sent to the review committee, they are evaluated against many different criteria. Readability is gauged using the Fry Readability Scale. Committee members look at layout issues, such as amount of white space and use of bulleted lists, use of medical jargon, and whether images support the main objective. For example, one document showed someone demonstrating an injection in a way that was not described in the text. Appropriateness of text is also examined. "We had a decontamination sheet that wasn't text-heavy, but it was terrifying," remembers Evans. "We rewrote it in a way that still conveyed the seriousness of what was happening but didn't frighten the patients."

Materials that do not meet the review criteria may be handled in a variety of ways. If the authors' meaning is clear, but language needs to be refined for readability, committee members may simply make the corrections

and send them back to the authors. For example, a recent consent form was revised to follow a question-and-answer format similar to the Ask Me 3 questions so information could be presented more clearly. If more extensive changes are required, reviewers may go back to the department where the piece originated and talk about possible solutions.

The committee has also tried to make things easier for authors up-front. For example, having realized the number of consent forms that are generated by the research department and the complexity of issues that need to be covered, committee members took one of these forms and revised it from beginning to end using plain language and health literacy principles. This consent form is now given to new authors of research products to use as a guide for creating their own forms.

When pieces are sent to the Cultural Competence staff for translation, they are reviewed again for both the technical aspects of translation and the cultural appropriateness of materials—vocabulary, images, and so on—for the target audiences. "There may be individual issues with languages," says Tong. "If a term doesn't exist in Russian, we have to do something a little bit different for that translation. Or if a term is derogatory, we change

Figure 4-15. Pamphlet to Help Staff Create Patient-Friendly Materials

Cultural Awareness

Think of your audience

- **Consider culture and religion**
  - When possible, include staple foods that can be used as possible alternatives to American foods.
  - Consider gender roles and their impact on health care.
  - Consider religious observances and diets, notions of appropriateness, modesty, sexual taboos, etc.
  - Choose images carefully—they are not universal
  - Depict members of the community.

Does it translate?

- **Avoid expressions that cannot be translated or are "too American."** Idiomatic or popular expressions such as "Where's the beef?" or "brown bag lunch" may be difficult or impossible to translate. Try to avoid references to American history, sports, popular culture.
- **Size matters:** Translation can increase text length, expanding text up to 20%, sometimes forcing the use of font sizes that are nearly illegible. Try to keep your original text as brief and to the point as possible.

Document Creation and Review:

The Process

1. Create your document.
2. Have your department head review and approve the document.
3. Submit the document to External Affairs for literacy review, branding and translation.
4. You may be contacted with questions about your document.
5. Receive your completed, totally fabulous document and start giving it to your patients!

External Affairs Department
Kathy Johannesen   Neal Gorman
718-630-8852   718-630-8316
kjohannesen@lmcmc.com   ngorman@lmcmc.com

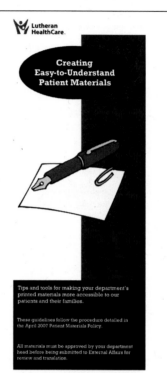

Lutheran HealthCare.

Creating Easy-to-Understand Patient Materials

Tips and tools for making your department's printed materials more accessible to our patients and their families.

These guidelines follow the procedure detailed in the April 2007 Patient Materials Policy.

All materials must be approved by your department head before being submitted to External Affairs for review and translation.

The Writing Process

PLAIN LANGUAGE

Organization
- Divide your text under clarifying headings. Keep sections brief.
- Emphasize and summarize main points.

Style
- Use everyday words.
- Explain technical terms and use examples.
- Avoid long, complex sentences.
- Avoid the passive voice. For example, instead of "The patient will be given a prescription by the physician," say "We will give you a prescription."
- Engage the reader. For example, use a question and answer format
- Explain useful, realistic steps the patient can take
- Make sure that cultural references are appropriate

TYPE AND SPACING

- Use a readable type style.
  - A footed or 'serif' font (this one is called "Rockwell") is most readable.
  - Use a 12– to 14-point font size.
- Use appropriate space between lines (generally 1.2 to 1.5 spacing).
- Do not print words on dark or patterned background.
- Use upper and lower case; avoid all cap text.
- Include ample white space.
- Leave right margin jagged.
- Do not split words across two lines.

OVERALL DESIGN

- Use graphics that are culturally relevant and contribute to your message.
- Avoid clutter.
- Clearly label all illustrations and charts.
- Use consistent and easily recognized headings.
- Signal main points with bold or highlights.

REVIEW PROCESS

- Review all materials and use a consistent check list.
- Use the readability check in MSWord.
- Engage members of the intended audience in a critical review process.
- Re-work the materials based on these reviews.

Source: Lutheran HealthCare. Used with permission.

This handout helps remind staff of important considerations for writing and designing patient materials that are useful for all audiences.

that. For example, *stroke centers* are bad things in the Chinese language; Chinese people wouldn't go there. So we call it a *neurological center*."

Materials in both English and other languages are often pilot tested in Lutheran HealthCare's adult education classes. The students in these classes are the same as the system's patient population, so staff get immediate, helpful feedback.

Building on Successes

Because the process is still being implemented, quantitative data collection to measure the impact has not yet been initiated. However, the staff have seen some positive outcomes. "We've actually had an increase in patient use of certain programs, such as rehabilitation," says Johannesen. "We took one brochure with four or five different topics and converted it to rack cards for each topic. A rack card is a one-page (front and back) brochure that gives concise information. These cards gave people enough information to get them to call in, which gave the health center staff the opportunity to sell their services. We saw an increase in business in each of the areas addressed by the rack cards."

Looking back at the journey they've made so far, committee members agree that there are things they might do differently and things they would like to improve on. For example, because the same types of health literacy issues were identified over and over during the initial binder review, it might have been sufficient to sample a few materials from each department rather than all of them. In addition, based on the print pieces they currently see, they have also advocated for increased training to make more of the system's authors aware of the need for better communication tools.

The committee is also looking for ways to streamline the review process. Many departments that do send materials for review do not anticipate the length of time it takes to get through three departments, and they push for shorter turnaround times to meet deadlines for special events and other needs. Improving the initial writing process would also help to move pieces through review more quickly, so committee members are exploring ways to make templates and samples available to authors on the system intranet or through another mechanism.

The overall goal is to craft products that are helpful and meaningful to the patients who will try to use them. As Lennon notes, "It's not just about someone's reading level, it's about communicating well."

APPENDIX

HEALTH LITERACY RESOURCES

The following list of resources is not meant to be exhaustive, but it will give you a starting point for your own health literacy research. Entries in each section are alphabetized by organization or tool name.

General Information and Comprehensive Sites

Agency for Healthcare Research and Quality (AHRQ)
http://www.ahrq.gov/browse/hlitix.htm
The Health Literacy and Cultural Competency page of the AHRQ's Web site includes links to agency press releases, patient resources, evidence reports (*see* later section for two examples), quality tools, and guidelines.

American Medical Association (AMA) Foundation
http://www.ama-assn.org/ama/pub/about-ama/
our-people/affiliated-groups/ama-foundation.shtml
The AMA Foundation gives general background information on health literacy on its Web site. There are links to articles and publications such as *Improving Communication—Improving Care* and *An Ethical Force Program Consensus Report,* as well as other literacy-related Web sites. Perhaps most useful is the variety of tool kits, instructional videos, tip cards, brochures, and other materials for health literacy programs available.

California Health Literacy Initiative
http://www.cahealthliteracy.org
This site can provide you with health literacy research and policies for the state and the nation. The initiative's online resource library provides articles and other resources, as well as sources for easy-to-read health information.

Harvard School of Public Health (HSPH)
http://www.hsph.harvard.edu/healthliteracy
On this extensive site from the Health Literacy Studies division of HSPH, you can find research and policy

reports; health literacy curricula for adult, medical school, and public health education; guides for assessing and creating written patient materials; and a huge list of related Web sites. You can also download the full text of the second edition of Doak, Doak, and Root's classic text *Teaching Patients with Low Literacy Skills* (http://www.hsph.harvard.edu/healthliteracy/doak.html).

The Joint Commission
http://www.jointcommission.org
Here, you can download copies of the Hospitals, Language, and Culture (HLC) research reports *Exploring Cultural and Linguistic Services in the Nation's Hospitals* and *One Size Does Not Fit All: Meeting the Health Care Needs of Diverse Populations.* They describe the challenges faced by a cross-section of hospitals across the nation in trying to serve patients of different cultures and make recommendations for ways to meet these challenges. Chapter 8 in the second report includes a self-assessment tool you can use to evaluate your organization's infrastructure, its data collection and use, and its methods for addressing cultural diversity. The white paper *What Did the Doctor Say? Improving Health Literacy to Protect Patient Safety* is also available.

Brochures and other materials for the Speak Up™ initiative can be downloaded at http://www.jointcommission.org/GeneralPublic/Speak+Up.

Medical Library Association (MLA)
http://mlanet.org/resources/healthlit
The health information literacy page for the MLA features links to resources for health care professionals and consumers. Topics include the MLA's Health Information Literacy Project, communicating with older adults, and health literacy in adult education.

National Literacy and Health Program, Canadian Public Health Association

http://www.cpha.ca/en/portals/h-l.aspx

This site has links to fact sheets and statistics; suggested strategies and solutions to poor health literacy; and tools, resources, and services.

Office of Disease Prevention and Health Promotion

http://www.health.gov/communication/literacy/default.htm

This division of the U.S. Department of Health & Human Services' Web site provides links to research and reports, government resources, and tools for improving health literacy such as sample action plans for health care organizations.

Office of Minority Health

http://www.omhrc.gov

If you search this site for "health literacy," you will find a long list of links to journal articles, committee reports, grants and programs, and patient education tools.

Partnership for Clear Health Communication at the National Patient Safety Foundation

http://www.npsf.org/pchc

The home page for this nonprofit coalition includes information on becoming a partner, links to pertinent press releases and newsletters, and links to downloads for policy reports and research.

Pfizer Clear Health Communication Initiative

http://www.pfizerhealthliteracy.com

This Web site has sections aimed at public health professionals, policymakers and researchers, media, and physicians and other providers. The latter section includes general information on health literacy; downloads of the Newest Vital Sign and Prevalence Calculator for screening, as well as various tools for improving written and verbal communication; information on grants and partnerships; a health literacy quiz to let you determine how much you actually know about the subject; and links to reports and research on health literacy.

World Education

http://healthliteracy.worlded.org/index.htm

This Health and Literacy Special Collection contains sections for health educators, teachers, and new readers. You can find facts and statistics about health literacy, policies and legislation, and online discussions here. The "Health Educators" section includes links to various initiatives, easy-to-read and multilingual health information, graphics-based materials and Web sites, information on cultural competence, and research.

Reports and Research

Agency for Healthcare Research and Quality (AHRQ)

http://www.ahrq.gov/downloads/pub/evidence/pdf/literacy/literacy.pdf

You can download the complete 2004 *Literacy and Health Outcomes* report from this site. If you just want a summary of the report, it is available at http://www.ahrq.gov/clinic/epcsums/litsum.htm.

http://healthit.ahrq.gov

On this main page, click on "Health IT Tools," then on "Health IT Literacy Guide" to find *Accessible Health Information Technology (IT) for Populations with Limited Literacy: A Guide for Developers and Purchasers of Health IT*. It gives ideas and a checklist for developers and purchasers of technology who want to make that technology accessible to all users.

The Commonwealth Fund

http://www.commonwealthfund.org

If you use the keywords "health literacy" to search this site, you will find myriad reports and research on topics covering best practices, outcomes of low health literacy, informed consent, improving care through improved health literacy, and many others.

Educational Testing Service

http://www.ets.org

This site has several key reports, such as *America's Perfect Storm: Three Forces Changing Our Nation's Future* (2007), *Literacy and Health in America* (2004), and *The Twin Challenges of Mediocrity and Inequality: Literacy in the U.S. from an International Perspective* (2002).

Institute of Medicine (IOM)

http://www.iom.edu/?id=19750

You can order a copy of the IOM's *Health Literacy: A Prescription to End Confusion* report here.

Language Services Action Kit

http://www.cmwf.org/usr_doc/LEP_actionkit_reprint_0204.pdf

You can download or print out this report developed by the Access Project and the National Health Law Program. It explains federal laws and policies about ensuring access to health care services for people with limited English proficiency, discusses how states can get federal funding to help pay for such services, describes state models for reimbursing health care organizations for language services, and suggests steps for advocating the need for these services.

National Center for Education Statistics

http://nces.ed.gov/naal

This Web site gives details about the 2003 National Assessment of Adult Literacy, including how it was developed and administered, key findings, and sample questions.

National Institute for Literacy

http://www.nifl.gov

A search for "health literacy" will take you to a list of reports and discussions of how health literacy can be incorporated into adult education courses.

Robert Wood Johnson Foundation

http://www.rwjf.org

If you search for "health literacy" on this site, you will find a large selection of research and policy reports, press releases, grant results, and journal articles.

Tools

Administration on Aging

http://www.aoa.gov/AoARoot/AoA_Programs/Tools_Resources/Older_Adults.aspx

This site provides links to resources for improving communication with and the health literacy of older adults. The links cover general communication principles,

health literacy, the use of plain language, and guidelines for designing Web sites.

Adult Literacy Estimates

https://www.casas.org/lit/litcode/search.cfm

This site allows you to search for estimates of adult literacy in a specific state, county, city/town, or congressional district.

Agency for Healthcare Research and Quality Pharmacy Tools

http://www.ahrq.gov/qual/pharmlit

Here you will find the download of *Is Our Pharmacy Meeting Patients' Needs? A Pharmacy Health Literacy Assessment Tool User's Guide.* You can also obtain a print copy by calling the AHRQ Publications Clearinghouse at 800/358-9295 or e-mailing ahrqpubs@ahrq.hhs.gov.

http://www.ahrq.gov/qual/pharmlit/pharmtrain.htm

This is the place to find the free materials comprising *Strategies to Improve Communication Between Pharmacy Staff and Patients: A Training Program for Pharmacy Staff.*

American Cancer Society (ACS)

http://www.cancer.org

The society's National Cancer Information Center has two versions of its information about major cancer types. The first is comprehensive and is intended for people with high health literacy; the second provides a synopsis of the same material written in plain language at an eighth-grade reading level.

http://www.cancer.org/docroot/PRO/content/PRO_3_Easy_Reading_Health_information.asp

This section of the ACS's Web site lets you download easy-to-read information about the importance of colorectal screening, smoking cessation, mammograms, Pap smears, and prostate testing. The information is available in 15 languages, including Arabic, Korean, Chinese, Hindi, Urdu, Polish, Bengali, and Russian.

Ask Me 3™

http://www.npsf.org/askme3

This is the site to visit for a full explanation of the Ask Me 3 intervention—its purpose, how to use it, and downloads of patient brochures (in several languages) and posters.

Center for Plain Language

http://centerforplainlanguage.org

This site offers guidelines for creating plain language materials, a tool kit for promoting plain language in your organization, and other tips on simplifying communication.

Centers for Disease Control and Prevention

http://www.cdc.gov/od/oc/simpput.pdf

This guide can help you make complicated and/or scientific information easier for all users to understand and identify with.

Consumer Health Vocabulary Initiative

http://consumerhealthvocab.org

You can use the tool on this site to find alternative words and phrases for medical jargon. You may also recommend the site to patients, who can use it to help "decode" information they may find elsewhere.

Expecting the Best

http://www.expectingthebest.org

The site for North Carolina's statewide effort to include health literacy in adult education has details on the project's background, an overview of the curriculum, suggestions for implementing similar programs, and links to health literacy resources. You will also find instructions for how to purchase the 14-lesson curriculum, an instructor's manual, and student lessons on a CD-ROM.

Hablamos Juntos

http://www.hablamosjuntos.org/signage/symbols/default.using_symbols.asp

This site has a library of universal symbols developed for signage in health care organizations. In addition to the library of symbols, you can download a workbook of best practices for using symbols, reports on how the symbols were developed, and supplemental symbols from the Department of Transportation.

Health Resources and Services Administration (HRSA)

http://www.hrsa.gov/servicedelivery/language.htm

This page of the HRSA's Web site gives plain language principles and a thesaurus to help you improve the readability of Health Insurance Portability and Accountability Act (HIPAA) privacy notices.

Healthy People 2010

http://odphp.osophs.dhhs.gov/projects/HealthComm

Although you can find general information about the Healthy People 2010 initiative at http://www.healthypeople.gov, the site listed here lets you download the Office of Disease Prevention and Health Promotion's action plans for improvement of health literacy.

Healthy Roads Media

http://www.healthyroadsmedia.org

This Web site provides a selection of audio, video, multimedia, and written materials on topics ranging from chronic diseases such as asthma and cancer to smoking and nutrition. The downloads are available in 19 languages, including Amharic, Burmese, Farsi, French, Hmong, Korean, Russian, and Somali.

LaRue Medical Literacy Exercises

http://mcedservices.com/medex/medex.htm

Created by Charles LaRue with a grant from the Minnesota Department of Children, Families and Learning, this Web site allows you to refer patients to the interactive online learning modules or to print out the learning materials for use in face-to-face education. The lessons cover interpreting prescription and over-the-counter labels, special warning labels, and side effects of medications. Both the interactive and print versions are available in English, Arabic, Hmong, Somali, and Spanish.

MedlinePlus®

http://www.nlm.nih.gov/medlineplus

This site is an excellent resource for your patients to

find easy-to-read information on diseases and conditions, drugs and supplements, testing, and other health topics in a wide variety of languages. There is also a medical encyclopedia and dictionary to help them interpret information from other sources and interactive tutorials with audio on many topics (http://www.nlm.nih.gov/medlineplus/tutorial.html). Guidelines for writing easy-to-read materials are provided at http://www.nlm.nih.gov/medlineplus/etr.html.

National Cancer Institute

http://www.nci.nih.gov/cancerinformation/clearandsimple

This Web site gives you a step-by-step guide to creating effective print materials for people with low literacy. Appendixes give ideas for layout, visual and multimedia aids, content, and other resources.

National Center for the Study of Adult Learning and Literacy (NCSALL)

http://www.ncsall.net/?id=1163

This is the main page for downloading sections of the NCSALL's guide *The Health Literacy Environment of Hospitals and Health Centers. Partners for Action: Making Your Healthcare Facility Literacy-Friendly.* It is aimed at leaders and health care staff and gives suggestions for analyzing and meeting the needs of your patient population. Training materials on related topics such as health care access and navigation, chronic disease management, and disease prevention are also available.

National Institute on Aging (NIA)'s Alzheimer's Disease Education & Referral (ADEAR) Center

http://www.alzheimers.nia.nih.gov

Check here for information about and to order copies of the NIA's free booklets *Understanding Memory Loss* and *Understanding Alzheimer's Disease.* You can also call 800/438-4380.

National Quality Forum (NQF)

http://www.qualityforum.org/pdf/reports/informed_consent_guide.pdf

This is the place to download a copy of the NQF's guide for *Implementing a National Voluntary Consensus*

Standard for Informed Consent, which presents a way to improve the informed consent process by using teach-back and the NQF's Safe Practice 10.

NIHSeniorHealth

http://nihseniorhealth.gov

If your practice or organization works with older patients, this Web site can be a good resource to recommend. Developed by the National Institute on Aging and the National Library of Medicine, it allows users to make text larger for easier viewing. Information is presented in an easy-to-read format, and navigation is straightforward.

Plain Language: Improving Information from the Federal Government to the Public

http://plainlanguage.gov

Although originally developed for use with government publications, the tools and tips on this site can help you simplify your own written materials.

Rapid Estimate of Adult Literacy in Medicine (REALM)

You can purchase copies of the REALM testing materials, which include laminated patient word lists, scoring sheets, and the administration manual, by contacting Terry Davis, Ph.D., Department of General Internal Medicine, P.O. Box 33932, Shreveport, LA 71130; phone: 318/675-4584; e-mail: tdavis1@lsumc.edu. Be sure to specify whether you want the adult version in regular or large font or the Rapid Estimate of Adolescent Literacy in Medicine (REALM-Teen).

Refugee Health Information Network

http://rhin.org

Refugee health professionals have created this site to give people from other countries health information in a variety of languages and to provide other professionals with information and tools for assessing and communicating with these patients. There is also a separate section on available health services specifically for refugees.

Rhode Island Health Literacy Project
http://www.rihlp.org/pubs/Complete_toolkit_224pgs.pdf
This tool kit, designed for physicians and providers, addresses health literacy, advance directives, palliative care, and cultural competency. It includes communication tips, sample forms, and lists of resources.

SALUD: Spanish Access to Literature/Uso Directo
http://palantir.lib.uic.edu/salud
The Web site for the SALUD project contains patient education materials in English and Spanish selected by the Chicago Department of Public Health in collaboration with the University of Illinois at Chicago Library of Health Sciences and College of Nursing.

SMOG (Simple Measure of Gobbledygook) Readability Calculator
http://www.harrymclaughlin.com/SMOG.htm
You can find the different readability formulas on many Web sites. This site features the SMOG creator's original formula; you can type in 30 to 2,000 words and have the calculator estimate the grade level.

Test of the Functional Health Literacy in Adults (TOFHLA)
To purchase TOFHLA testing materials, including the original and short English and Spanish versions in standard and large fonts, along with directions for use, contact Peppercorn Books & Press, P.O. Box 693, Snow Camp, NC 27349; phone: 336/376-6935; fax: 336/376-9099; e-mail: post@peppercornbooks.com; Web site: http://www.peppercornbooks.com.

U.S. Food and Drug Administration (FDA)
http://www.fda.gov/opacom/lowlit/7lowlit.html
You can print out PDF files or order printed brochures for English and Spanish populations on this Web site. Written in an easy-to-read format using simple terms, the wide range of topics includes arthritis, diabetes, eating well, disease prevention, feeding infants, and hearing loss.

U.S. Pharmacopeia (USP)
http://www.usp.org/audiences/consumers/pictograms
You can download the 81 USP pictograms available on this Web site in .gif or .eps format after signing the license agreement. The pictograms are standardized graphic images that you can use to help explain medication instructions, precautions, and/or warnings to patients.

YOU: The Smart Patient: An Insider's Handbook for Getting the Best Treatment, by Michael F. Roizen, M.D., and Mehmet C. Oz, M.D., with The Joint Commission
This book uses humor and whimsical illustrations to provide concrete guidance to patients in navigating the health care system and getting involved in their own health care. Popular authors Roizen and Oz show readers in clear, easy steps how to take control of their own health care. Of particular note is an appendix explaining medical jargon. You can order copies of the book at The Joint Commission's Web site, http://www.jcrinc.com/YOU-The-Smart-Patient, or by calling 877/223-6866.

Training

Health Resources and Services Administration (HRSA)
http://hrsa.gov/healthliteracy/training.htm
This division of the U.S. Department of Health & Human Services offers free online training for public health professionals in a course called United Health Communication 101: Addressing Health Literacy, Cultural Competence, and Limited English Proficiency. The course may be taken for continuing education credit and requires approximately five hours to complete.

University of Virginia Health System School of Medicine
http://healthsystem.virginia.edu/internet/som-hlc
The information and tools found here can help you develop a health literacy curriculum.

World Education
http://www.worlded.org/WEIInternet
Search "health literacy" on this Web site to find a list of U.S. and international programs that exist to promote better health and literacy levels.

GLOSSARY

Audience-centered communications – Communications that are tailored to meet the literacy and learning needs of targeted segments of the public

Client-centered communications – Communications that are tailored to meet the literacy and learning needs of health plan enrollees

ESL – English as a Second Language

National Standards on Culturally and Linguistically Appropriate Services (CLAS) – A set of 14 guidelines established in 2001 by the U.S. Department of Health & Human Services' Office of Minority Health. Directed at health care organizations and individual providers, the standards exist to help them make their services more accessible to all populations.

Health information – Any information, oral or recorded in any form or medium, that is created by a health care provider, health plan, public health authority, employer, life insurer, school or university, or health care clearinghouse, and which relates to the past, present, or future physical or mental health or condition, the provision of health care, or payment for the provision of health care to an individual

Health literacy – 1. The ability to obtain, process, and understand basic health information and services needed to make appropriate health decisions and follow instructions for treatment (Institute of Medicine [IOM] and the American Medical Association [AMA]) 2. The degree to which individuals have the capacity to obtain, process, and understand basic health information and services needed to make appropriate decisions (National Library of Medicine, Healthy People 2010 [http://www.healthypeople.gov] and the American College of Physicians (ACP) Foundation)

Informed consent – Agreement or permission accompanied by full notice about the care, treatment, or service that is the subject of the consent. A patient must be apprised of the nature, risks, and alternatives

of a medical procedure or treatment before the physician or other health care professional begins any such course. After receiving this information, the patient then either consents to or refuses such a procedure or treatment.

Jargon – Specialized language of a trade, profession, or similar group

LEP – Limited English proficient

Mental health literacy – A person's knowledge and beliefs about mental illness

Maternal health literacy – Cognitive and social skills that determine the motivation and ability of women to gain access to, understand, and use information in ways that promote and maintain their health and that of their children*

Patient-centered communications – Communications that are tailored to meet the literacy and learning needs of the individual patient

REALM – Rapid Estimate of Adult Literacy in Medicine; a word recognition test in which patients are asked to read aloud a series of words and terms commonly used in clinical settings

Repeat back – Method to ensure understanding of information being communicated, often used between members of a care-giving team, by asking the receiver of the information to "repeat back" what was said

Readability formulas/scales – Math-based procedures (often computerized) that use word and sentence length to identify the grade level at which text is written. They are used to help determine how much simplification the language and writing style of a piece may require.

---

* Renkert S., Nutbeam D.: Opportunities to improve maternal health literacy through antenatal education: An exploratory study. *Health Promot Int* 16(4):381–388, 2001.

The Flesch-Kincaid Grade Level and Gunning FOG Index are two examples of these.

Show back – A method to ensure understanding of information being communicated, often used between a caregiver and a patient, by asking the receiver of the information to demonstrate, or "show back" what was demonstrated

Teach back – A method to ensure understanding of information being communicated, often used between a caregiver and a patient, by asking the receiver of the information to "teach back" what was said

TOFHLA – Test of Functional Health Literacy in Adults; a functional literacy assessment tool used to test patients' reading comprehension and numeracy skills using actual materials from health care settings

Universal precautions – An approach meaning that all discussions and materials are simple enough for everyone to understand, regardless of literacy level

INDEX

A

ACP (American College of Physicians) Foundation, 2, 14
ACRIA (AIDS Community Research Initiative of America), 15
ACS. *See* American Cancer Society (ACS)
Action plan for improving health literacy (ODPHP), 38, 39–40
ADEAR (Alzheimer's Disease Education & Referral) Center, 123
Administration on Aging, 121
Adult education, 17
Adult Literacy Estimates, 121
Adult literacy levels, 4–5, 6
Adverse events and medical errors
    communication and, 9
    health literacy and, v, 5, 24
Agency for Healthcare Research and Quality (AHRQ)
    National Health Literacy Act of 2007 (S. 2424), 10, 12
    pharmacy staff literacy tools, 12, 73, 121
    resources, 119, 120, 121
    statistics on health literacy, 1
AIDS Community Research Initiative of America (ACRIA), 15
Alzheimer's Disease Education & Referral (ADEAR) Center, 123
AMA. *See* American Medical Association (AMA)
AMA Foundation. *See* American Medical Association (AMA) Foundation
Ambulatory care organizations, 34
Ambulatory patients, 24
American Cancer Society (ACS), 5, 121
    National Cancer Information Center, 15, 121
American College of Physicians (ACP) Foundation
    health literacy definition, 2
    Health Literacy Solutions Program, 14
    Patient Literacy Program Focus Policy, 14
American Medical Association (AMA)
    Code of Medical Ethics, 13
    English language skills, report on, 22
    Ethical Force Program, 14
    health literacy definition, 1
    health literacy improvements, support for, 17
American Medical Association (AMA) Foundation
    health literacy initiatives, 13–14
    health literacy training, 41
    Health Literacy Train-the-Trainer program, 13, 83, 89
    Helping Your Patients Understand, 64
    resources, 119
American Pharmaceutical Association, 15
American Society of Health-System Pharmacists, 15
America's Perfect Storm (Educational Testing Service), 4–5
Appointment procedures, 38, 41
Ask Me 3™ program, 14, 43, 46–47, 64–68, 84–87, 121–122
    case studies, 65–67, 68, 80, 84–85, 86
Assessment of health literacy
    basis for, 25
    behaviors that hide poor literacy level, 25
    demographics of high-risk and vulnerable populations, 21–24
        age, 21, 22
        education and income, 21–22
        English proficiency, 21, 22–23
        race and culture, 21, 23
    discussion techniques, 25–26
    misconceptions about at-risk patients, 24–25
    population-level information, 32–33

standardized assessment tools, 26–32
    Literacy Assessment for Diabetes, 31
    Newest Vital Sign, 14, 29, 32
    Nutritional Literacy Test, 31
    REALM, 27, 29, 31–32, 123
    REALM-Short Form, 27
    REALM-Teen, 27
    SAHLSA, 32
    TOFHLA, 6, 27–28, 30–31, 124
    worksheet for selecting, 28
    WRAT-R3, 31

B

Basic health literacy, 2, 3, 4
Behavior choices, health literacy level and, 7
Behaviors that hide poor literacy level, 25
Bellevue Hospital Center case study, 105–111
Below basic health literacy, 3, 4
Bronson Healthcare Group case study, 62–69
Brown-bag medication reviews, 26

C

California Endowment, 10, 16
California Health Literacy Initiative, 13, 119
Canadian literacy survey, 5
Canadian Public Health Association, National Literacy and Health Program, 120
Cancer screenings, 7, 33
Care and treatment. *See also* Environment of care; Outcomes of care
    access to, 7–8
    costs of, 8, 21–22
    culturally competent care, 8–9, 10, 34
        CLAS standards, 11, 12
    emergency care, 7, 8
    empowering and encouraging participation in care, 42–44
        case studies, 65–69
    hospitalization rates, 7, 8
    media advertisements and information, impact of, 49
    principles for effective communication and, 9
    terminology and jargon, 46, 47, 52
    use of health services and health literacy, 7–8, 33
Case studies
    Bellevue Hospital Center, 105–111
    Bronson Healthcare Group, 62–69
    Emory University, 70–74
    Grady Health System, 75–82
    Iowa Health System, 83–88
    Lutheran HealthCare, 112–117
    Minnesota Alliance for Patient Safety, 89–104
    New York University School of Medicine, Bellevue Hospital Center, 105–111
Center for Plain Language, 122
Centers for Disease Control and Prevention (CDC), 122
Centers for Medicare & Medicaid Services (CMS)
    access to care through, 8
    Consumer Assessment of Healthcare Providers and Systems Hospital Survey (H-CAHPS), 87
    costs of health care, 8
    interpreter services, 44
    Medicare and Medicaid, health literacy and, 22